Becoming Miss Izzy

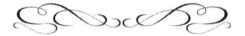

Sue Zook, Ed. D.

and

Mary Lazarski

Absolute Author Publishing House
New Orleans, LA

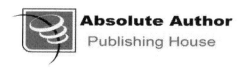

Absolute Author
Publishing House

Becoming Miss Izzy
Copyright © 2019 by Sue Zook

Publisher: Absolute Author Publishing House
Publishing Editor: Dr. Melissa Caudle
Copy Editor: Erin N. Wright
Associate Editor: Nancy Pile
Cover Designer: Jesh Arts Studio

Library of Congress Cataloging-in-Publication Data

Zook, Sue and Lazarski, Mary.

p.cm.

ISBN-13: 978-1-7337182-7-1

1. Nonfiction 2. Self-help 3. Weight 4. Anti-Bullying

---

0 1 2 3 4 5 6 7 8 9

Printed in the United States of America

TABLE OF CONTENTS

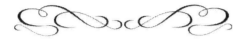

Introduction

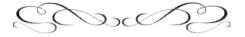

Let's imagine for a minute you wake up one morning and have magical superpowers that can transport you to another place and time. You can go back to the past or forward to the future. Just say the magic words, "Take me on an adventure," to make it happen.

Before you get too excited, you need to know that this superpower comes with a few strings attached.

The first condition is you can only use your superpower a single time. That's right, only once! And, you don't get to pick where you will end up. You might end up in the most amazing place of your wildest dreams. Where would that be? Worse, you might end up in some scary place alone.

What if your superpowers transport you to some future space galaxy? Or, an African safari, surrounded by man-eating tigers and lions? There's a chance you could end up in a life as you know it, in a different neighborhood, with a different family, or in a different state. You could sail the seven seas and visit exotic tropical islands. Your adventure might include a trip around the world with stops at every amusement park. You could end up riding every roller coaster invented. The possibilities are endless.

Here's another catch. You can't choose how long the adventure will last. It might be two hours, a few days, or even longer. Remember, you don't get to choose. The only guarantee is that it won't last longer than a year. How does that make you feel? It might be for a couple of hours. Could be a year from now.

Let me ask you—would you use your power? Is an unknown adventure worth taking a chance like that?

Today, I would say no way. But, what do I know? With my luck, I would end up somewhere like where I live now. Why bother? I live in a nice place. It's a suburban, middle-class neighborhood with lots of families. Homes are comfortable cookie-cutter houses, meaning they all look alike except for the different colors or types of flowers and decorations. The houses aren't too fancy like the ones in the town next door. The neighborhood is new, and our home has all the modern conveniences that most kids enjoy these days.

One of the nicest things about our neighborhood is the amazing park and field close to our house. I can walk just a few blocks and sit in a field filled with beautiful sunflowers. I love going there to be alone and sort through my thoughts and feelings in my head.

The little voice inside my head and a feeling I get in the pit of my stomach seem to say, "Don't use a superpower to end up on an unknown adventure."

What is that voice I sometimes hear? It seems to have to ask a lot of questions. Other times, it feels like it is trying to tell me what to do. Sometimes it's easy to pay attention to what I feel. Like today, I wouldn't use those magical powers. With my luck, I'd find myself in a creepy haunted house or worse. I'm convinced of that.

Besides, who needs superpowers anyway to have an adventure? Every day can be an adventure. You'll see what I mean.

My name is Elizabeth Ann Tanlin. OMG, what do you know, my initials spell EAT. Maybe that's why I'm FAT; or, at least I think I am fat. Maybe, I am chubbier than fat. I love to eat. My looks are average for a ten-year-old, fifth-grade girl. I wouldn't consider myself pretty, but I am not ugly either. My long hair is a reddish color in the fall but gets more strawberry-blonde when it gets kissed by the sun in the summer. I feel I am standing outside the crowd. That little voice and feeling I get seems to tell me I am too chubby.

When I was born, my mom said I was the most precious little thing; not fat by any means, weighing a little over seven pounds. I was a healthy and happy baby, according to my mom. How did I go from healthy and happy to thinking I am fat and feeling sad? This nagging voice and feeling I get makes me think a lot. Maybe even worry about things. It might be the worrying that makes me sad. It seems the closer it comes time to head to middle school, the more I worry, and the sadder I get.

I don't mean to keep bringing up my weight, but I think Elizabeth is a fat name. Do you? So, I like to have people call me Lizbeth or Liz or even Lizzy. Most people call me Lizbeth, except Momo, my grandma. She calls me Miss Izzy.

My mom is my Momo's daughter. She has told Momo over and over again not to call me, "Miss Izzy." Momo pays her no mind at all. She's called me that from the time I was old enough to walk, around the time I turned one. "Come to Momo, Miss Izzy," she would call out. And, I would toddle on over to Momo with my hands outstretched, ready for lifting and cuddling on her lap. I like that Momo still to this day calls me Miss Izzy.

I love my Momo to death. She is the coolest grandma that any kid could ask for in a grandmother. Even with her silvery-gray hair and the wrinkles on her face, I think my grandma is beautiful. She is super smart and always seems to know things. Sometimes when she asks a question, I don't have to say a word. Momo already knows the answer. She is kind, forgiving, and cares about people. If I'm feeling down or in one of my funky moods, Momo knows what to do to make things better. Even though she is getting old, at least when you are ten, most people in their sixties seem old, Momo is, what she likes to call, "young at heart." She still has fun and laughs a lot. Her good mood can be contagious. I hope when I get old, I can be like her.

My mom is the best. She is someone I admire -- my hero. Her name is Sarah Tanlin. Mom and I are close even though she is a busy, hardworking mom. She is a middle school principal. Thank God it's not at the school I will attend! Do you know how hard it is to have a principal for your mom? Think about it. You do something you don't want your mom to know about—you get caught. You try to give a lame excuse for something you shouldn't have done—she's heard it all. It's best if you follow the rules.

I wouldn't say my mom knows it all. She knows a little about almost everything. She takes after Momo that way. And, when she learns something new, she is bound to share it with others. What I like most about Mom is that she really does pay attention to and care about my feelings. When I don't understand why I'm feeling a certain way, I can count on Mom to set me straight and help me figure things out.

My dad, Rich Tanlin, is okay. I know that's not a very descriptive word. I'm sure you can think of a better one. It's not that I have any major problems with him. We get along most of the time, but he doesn't notice me or pay attention too much to what goes on in my life. Dad has his own business in sales. I don't understand it. He works from home, and you dare not bother him when he's in his office. I sometimes feel that Dad doesn't have a lot of interest in what is going on at home. He's all about work. Work, work, and more work for Dad. Except, he seems to take an interest in my brother, Joey.

Joey is eight years old. He is the big baby of the family. Joey's not fat or chubby, but he is sick a lot. From the time he was little, Mom was forever running him to the doctor. He always has colds or ear infections, and never sits still even when he's sick. He's got something the doctor calls ADHD. That's one reason he gets into trouble so much at school. My brother isn't mean like kids at school can be, but, he laughs at stuff when there is nothing funny going on, or blurts out comments in class when he shouldn't, or runs when he should walk, or makes a smart remark when it is not appropriate. Because of how he acts, he gets picked on. I don't like it when that happens. Mom calls his behavior impulsive. There's no excuse for kids to be mean.

Mean kids are another cause of worry for me. Heck, I don't like it when anybody gets picked on. I don't like it when it happens to Joey or any of my friends. That is for sure. I wish I had a superpower to stop all the meanness.

Rounding out the family are two adorable, three-year-old rescue dogs, Harmony and Hudson. They are brother and sister dogs, littermates they call it. And, we have a silly cat named Perkins. I love all three of them and couldn't imagine life without them.

So, let's pretend that you used your superpowers and ended up in my life. Come along and let me show you how anyone's life can be an adventure. Just turn the page to let the journey begin.

PART I

AWARENESS AND REALIZATION

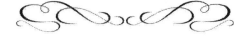

1. Am I Fat?

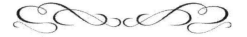

I asked without meeting my mom's eyes as I sat cross-legged on her bed, twirling the loose strands of her comforter with my fingers. "Am I fat?" She was sitting on a chair before a mirror, applying bronze makeup across her half-closed eye. I glanced up and caught her staring back at me in the mirror's reflection, her hand frozen in mid-swipe. She lowered her hand as the corners of her mouth turned up in a smile.

"Elizabeth," she started, "you've asked me this before."

As she turned in her chair to face me, I closed my eyes and thought of the first time I asked my mother this exact question.

I was eight years old and conflicted about which outfit to wear to my cousin's birthday party. I knew better than to ask Dad. His answer was always a bored, "You look fine," every time Mom asked the same questions. "Does this dress make me look fat?" "Do I still look pregnant?" "Are my legs too fat to wear shorts?" "Are these jeans too tight for my butt?" "Do you think I would be more attractive if I lost a few pounds?" "Should I get this top in a

SUE ZOOK AND MARY LAZARSKI

bigger size or a smaller size to make me look skinnier?" "Do I look fatter now with my hair cut shorter?"

I think Mom suspected that Dad wasn't being honest because she stopped asking him how she looked and asked me instead. How was I supposed to know the right answer? Moms are bigger than their kids, but just because she was bigger, taller, and older than me, didn't mean she was fat; did it? I was getting bigger, taller, and older too. Did that mean I was getting fat?

I remembered walking into my parent's bedroom wearing my first choice of outfit, a navy-blue dress with baby pink polka dots that ended just past my knees. I twirled, showing the dress off to my mom and repeated the question she'd asked me endless times. "Do I look fat in this?"

"Liz," Mom whispered, cradling her hand against my face, and bringing me back to the present. I opened my eyes and looked into hers, smiling at her half-painted eyelid. I wished with desperation for the same response she gave me when I was eight.

"You are *not* fat," she said. Softer, she continued, "You're my beautiful girl. The only concern you should have right now is getting your homework done tonight so we can have fun this weekend." She tickled my side, earning a chuckled response. "Now," she declared, "Go get started, so I can finish getting ready!" I jumped off her bed and ran for the door as she shooed me out of her room.

I stopped by my room to grab my math book and made my way downstairs to the kitchen. As I rummaged through the fridge looking for an orange Hi-C, my brother, Joey, bumped me against the door. Rattled, he knocked my hand aside and snatched the last juice box. Before I could protest, he stepped

3

back with a cocky smile that stretched his face like the Cheshire cat.

"Snooze you lose," he stated, obnoxiously slurping the juice.

"Hey, Dad," I called as he entered the kitchen. "Joey took the last Hi-C. Can I have a soda while I do my homework?"

Soda was off limits for us kids because of Joey's ADHD. "Too much caffeine," my parents would say. I always thought sugar amped him up. He always ran around like a banshee whenever he had a candy bar.

"Sure," Dad responded absently. He was pacing the kitchen and checking his watch, growing more impatient as each minute ticked by. "I don't understand why it takes hours to get ready," he grumbled under his breath.

I grabbed a soda from the fridge and smiled smugly at my brother as I popped the tab. "How's your juice?" I asked. *Ha! Jokes on you, brat-face!*

"Finally!" Dad exclaimed as Mom walked into the kitchen. "You realize we have a reservation, right?" he asked her as he swept the keys from the wall hook.

Mom looked at me expectantly as she turned in a circle, showcasing her style. "Well?" she asked hesitantly. "So, how do I look? Okay?"

I gave her a smile and two thumbs up. "You look great, Mom!" As she beamed from ear to ear, I wanted to change my initial words. She looked beautiful, always has.

2. Am I a Worrywart?

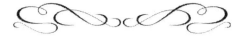

T he final bell rang, signaling school was over for the day. As I shoved my science book in my bag, Mr. Landry called me over to his desk. A few kids snickered as they left the classroom, no doubt thinking I was in trouble for something.

What now? I thought as I approached his desk.

"Hey there, Elizabeth," Mr. Landry started. "You don't have to look so worried!" he laughed. I shifted my bag to my other shoulder and took a deep breath, attempting to relieve the tension I felt.

"I only wanted to check in," he said concerned. "Noticed that you weren't present in class today. It looked like you were deep in thought," he said while tapping the side of his head, emphasizing his point. "Is everything okay?"

"I . . . I'm . . ." *I don't know!* As Mr. Landry waited for my response, I played with the buckle on my backpack. Open . . . close . .

. open . . . close, the click-clack noise filling the silent room. I glanced up to find my teacher smiling at me.

"Okay," I blew out the breath I was holding. "I'm nervous about middle school," I admitted. Feeling I could let my guard down, I continued, "I guess I've just been worrying about what it will be like. I think about it all the time."

Mr. Landry nodded his head in understanding. "Elizabeth, do you remember the seeds we planted in the little paper cups at the start of the school year?" he asked.

Wondering where this was going, I nodded my head as he continued, "Well, your worries are like the seed. Buried deep inside," he paused, "But if you don't express those feelings, eventually it will break the surface."

Realization hit me as I saw where he was going with this. "Like the little green sprout coming out of the soil?" I asked.

"Exactly!" Mr. Landry said and smiled. "Like the sprout, your worries will continue to grow bigger each day. Therefore, it's important to talk to someone about them."

I nodded my head in agreement. "Thanks, Mr. Landry, I will."

He smiled in response, then glanced at his watch. "You should get going; I'm sure your ride is outside waiting for you."

As I walked through the hallway, I thought about Mr. Landry's words and concern over me. *Am I the only kid that worries about things?* I was sure most kids wondered and worried about stuff too. Just like Mr. Landry, Mom and Momo thought I worried too much.

Anytime Momo would catch me daydreaming, or in a world of my own, she would sneak behind and wrap her arms around me, saying, "What are you thinking 'bout, Miss Izzy? Quit that worrying and go outside to play. You worrying about every little thing worries me."

As I passed through the large entry doors leading outside the school, I scanned the line of cars parked next to the curb, searching for a familiar one. My eyes were drawn to the one where a hand was waving through the sunroof. I laughed at how funny it looked to see Momo's wriggling fingers protruding from the top of the car.

"Miss Izzy!" Momo exclaimed as soon as I opened the car door. "Glad to see you made it outta there, honey. Seldom takes you that long once the final bell has rung." She raised her brow.

"Oh, well, Mr. Landry wanted to talk after class," I replied while snapping my seatbelt in place.

"And?" Momo waved me on.

"And," I sighed, "I guess Mr. Landry agrees with you and Mom." I let my words hang there, teasing my grandma.

Momo chuckled. "Well, Miss Izzy, any wise man would agree with us," she said, straightening herself in her seat.

We both dissolved in giggles.

"He thinks I worry too much and doesn't want me to keep it buried," I continued.

Momo nodded in agreement, saying, "A wise man, indeed."

3. Mindless Eater

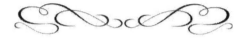

After Momo dropped me off at home, I found Joey sitting on the couch, snacking on sandwich cookies, and watching a silly show on the cartoon network. I sank into a spot next to him and sighed.

He glanced at me out of the corner of his eye and sighed himself. "What's up, Lizzy?" he asked.

I wanted to get outside. Let the sun warm me and feel the breeze flow through my hair. Listen to the birds chirping messages to one another. Feel the earthy grass tickle my feet and not think about a single thing.

"Can we go to the park until Mom and Dad get home?" I asked with my signature puppy-eyed look.

A groan escaped Joey. "Lizzy," he whined, "don't look at me like that. You know what happened last time." He cast his eyes down; sadness etched on his features. "Maybe Momo can take us to that big park in Riverside tomorrow." He stood up, abandoning his plate of cookies, and walked away.

Sitting alone in the living room, I heard his bedroom door open and then close. I wanted to run to his room and wrap him in a bear hug, but I knew better. He would need to be alone with his thoughts for a while before I attempted that. Even though he was a bratty jerk sometimes, he was still my brother, and I hated to see him so hurt.

My fingers found the stack of cookies my brother left behind. As I sat there eating, I thought back to that day in the park.

Joey and I were on the swing set, pumping our legs and trying to beat the other on how high we could go. It was my favorite game we played at the park even though Joey always won. As we slowed, laughing like a pair of hyenas, another boy approached the swings. Soon after, my brother's demeanor changed. He grew stiff and had an almost pained smile plastered on his face. I didn't know this boy, but it appeared my brother did.

When Joey's swing was low enough, the boy reached out and grabbed the chain, jerking my brother off his swing. The boy pointed at my brother who was struggling to stand and laughed. I watched wide-eyed, my jaw slack, as the boy continued to taunt Joey. He called him an "ugly dork" and some other terrible words Mom and Dad forbade us ever to say.

My brother didn't cry. Not in front of that mean boy. And, he didn't say a word. Didn't defend himself. Didn't call the boy mean names in return. He grabbed my hand, and we stormed out of the park.

It wasn't until later that evening, before I climbed into bed, that I could hear him sobbing in his room next to mine. I made a vow that night—if I ever saw that mean boy again, I would yell at him for treating Joey that way. I would stand up to bullies. They would never hurt him again, or me either.

I reached for another cookie, but my fingers hit an empty plate. *Did I eat all those cookies?* I hadn't been paying attention to anything other than my thoughts. Hoping Joey wouldn't choose this moment to exit his room and return for the cookies I ate, I scurried to the kitchen to throw away the evidence.

I was washing my hands in the kitchen sink when I heard the garage door opening. I grabbed my bag and pulled out my homework, saying a silent prayer it was Mom returning from work. I hadn't started my homework yet since I was preoccupied in a memory and scarfing down an entire plate of cookies.

A brief moment later, my mom walked through the kitchen door, and I breathed a sigh of relief. "Hi, honey," she said, her eyes buried in the mail she was sorting in her hands.

"Hi, Mom," I replied, waiting for her to look up at me. After leaving the mail in a stack on the counter, she turned in my direction. For a brief second, it worried me she would find a cookie crumb on my lip.

"I need to get a few things from the store before Joey's baseball game tonight," she said and then sighed. "Ready to go?"

I sprang up from the barstool, eager to go. I loved the Winn-Dixie supermarket and all the delicious little treats they offered for free!

SUE ZOOK AND MARY LAZARSKI

"What about Joey?" I asked, realizing he was still upstairs in his room.

"Your father will be home soon," she replied. "They will meet us at the game later."

It didn't take long to reach the supermarket -- one advantage of living in such a small town. As Momo would say, everything is just a "hop, skip, and jump" away. I laughed to myself while picturing my grandma hopping, skipping, and jumping her way around town.

As we stepped inside Winn-Dixie, the scents of roasted meat and oven-fresh baked bread welcomed me. I wanted to close my eyes and inhale, savoring the aroma, but Mom was on a mission, snagging a cart and power walking down the first aisle. I jogged to keep up with her but stopped at the end of the aisle when I noticed the first sample table.

"Hey, darlin,' want to try a new product?" the lady at the booth beckoned me over, enticing me with a little paper cup full of what looked like chocolate goo. At least I hoped it was chocolate.

I wandered to the booth and peered into the cup she handed me. Before I could ask, she mentioned it was dark fudge pudding made by some farm a couple of miles down the road. If enough people liked it, they would sell it in the store.

I took a tentative taste, a tiny little speck on my spoon, just to make sure it was chocolate and not cow poo. It was made at a farm, so what did I know? The best-tasting pudding ever was a reward to my taste buds. I lapped up the rest of my cup in record time.

The lady smiled, knowing by my reaction that the pudding was amazing. "You should sell this here!" I exclaimed. "It's so good! I bet my brother…"

I was cut off by my mom, who yelled across the store, "Elizabeth!"

I threw my little cup in the waste bin next to the booth and waved goodbye to the sample lady. As I made my way across the store to Mom, I passed another booth. This one had samples of different olives. Gross! Olives were the grossest-tasting things on this planet. I was happy to skip that booth.

I spotted Mom at the deli counter squinching her fingers to show the man she wanted the meat sliced paper-thin. I figured I had a little more time to explore, so I shuffled my way near the frozen food aisle. A line of booths offering more samples waited to surprise me as I turned the corner. I tried pizza squares, brownie bites, lemon tortes, juice pouches, fruit snacks, and fried cheese curds; all super yummy. I hoped that next time we visited Winn-Dixie, those sample products would be stocked and ready to buy.

After loading the bags into the car, Mom mentioned how starved she was. As she was rambling on about how you should never go grocery shopping hungry, I felt my swollen stomach and realized I'd already eaten my dinner in samples. Not to mention that plate of cookies I had earlier.

"Ooh, I know!" Mom said, turning with a smile. "Let's grab burgers to-go from Mickey's and eat at the game! I know it's your fave!"

I wanted to groan. I didn't think I could fit anything else in. However, seeing the goofy smile on Mom's face had me shaking my head in approval. I knew she was hungry, and I didn't want to disappoint her.

One Mickey burger and some curly fries later, I felt like I would burst. I tried to focus on Joey's baseball game, but my grumbling stomach wouldn't let me. I was miserably sandwiched between Mom and Dad on the bleachers. Worse was the time I spent in the bathroom hugging the toilet. I hate throwing up. It's a good note to self not to stuff myself to the gills.

Mom had to nudge me awake when we arrived home. Before crawling up the stairs and flopping into bed, I asked Mom who'd won the baseball game. I should have known the answer. Joey's team always lost.

4. Mom's Mini-Me

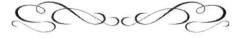

My eyes opened to slits as I awoke by feeling a cold and wet sensation on my hand, followed by a rumbling vibration near my side. I lifted my head and saw Perkins, our family cat, kneading the comforter. When he noticed me watching him, he trotted closer and gave a soft little chirp in greeting. He pressed his cold nose to my hand and nudged it for pets. I sank my fingers into his soft fur and closed my eyes, his contented purr luring me back to sleep.

The serene feeling didn't last long, however. I jolted awake as Hudson and Harmony barked in unison, alerting everyone in the house it was their breakfast time. That, or they had to go pee!

I groaned as I dragged myself from the bed and shuffled my way downstairs to see what the ruckus was. When I made my way into the kitchen, Mom was preparing the dog's breakfast. Their tails whipping against the cabinets as they stared in complete concentration as Mom scraped the sides of their food can.

"Mornin," I mumbled while rubbing my tired eyes. I hated those little crusty things that gathered in the corners after sleep. When I could focus again, I glanced at Harmony and Hudson. The two dogs always covered me in sloppy kisses every morning. To my disappointment, they didn't even look at me for fear of missing out on their meal preparation.

I must have made a face because Mom laughed. "Good morning, sweetie," she said grinning. "Harmony and Hudson act like they are starving this morning!" She set the bowls on the mat, and both dogs lunged for the food as if it were a competition. "I'm sure you'll get your morning kisses when they finish eating."

I slumped into the closest chair, stretching my legs as far as I could under the table. "What are we doing today?" I asked yawning.

Mom had just finished washing her hands in the sink and was drying them when she looked at the patio door. Following her gaze, it surprised me to see rain pelting the glass at a sharp angle. I sat up and jogged to the window, in disbelief of the pools of water gathering in patches around the yard.

"It's raining cats and dogs out there," she sighed. "And I have to take Joey to the doctor."

Joey almost lived at the doctor's office. He was always sick: ear and sinus infections, stomach pains, headaches, and bronchitis. It wouldn't surprise me if Dr. Adams had a bed and shower at his office just for Joey. Throw in an Xbox and some games, and we would never see him again!

"What's wrong with him now?" I whispered as I heard my brother's heavy feet stomping down the stairs. He let out a groan with each step he took as if it pained him. I rolled my eyes at his theatrics when Mom mouthed that he had another ear infection.

"Mooooom," Joey whined as he reached the kitchen doorway. "It hurts . . . sooooo bad." His whimpering and tears set Mom into motion. He was an outstanding performer.

I crossed my arms in front of my chest, leveling him with a look that said I didn't believe his act.

"It hurts, Elizabeth!" he snapped, glaring at me.

I relaxed my stance, shrugging my shoulders.

Mom, being the mediator, told my brother to wait in the car. "Don't worry, honey. I'm sure Dr. Adams will give you something to clear it up, and you'll feel much better," she reassured him.

After Joey left the room, Mom turned in my direction. "Your father is doing work in his office, so try not to disturb him," she warned.

I nodded my head. I knew better than to do that.

"There's Pop-Tarts or cereal in the cabinet if you want breakfast," she continued while snatching her keys off the counter. "I'll bring us home something for lunch after Joey's appointment. You should get a start on that report for school," she hinted as she gave a little wave before opening the door leading to the garage.

I'd forgotten all about that report! Grabbing my backpack, I pulled out my social studies folder containing the assignment. The report had to be something about "Life on the Frontier, A Glimpse of Western Civilization." I sighed as I walked to the cabinet, searching for the Pop-Tarts Mom mentioned. Shouldn't conduct research on an empty stomach!

While munching on the strawberry-flavored pastry, I remembered doing a report last year on horses. I figured since they had horses during the frontier period, I could use some of

16

that to start my report. It was their only means of transportation in the Wild West! Excited at the prospect of not having to start an essay from scratch, I finished my breakfast and started the hunt for my old report.

When searching my room was a bust, I turned to the basement. We kept bunches of old stuff down there. Maybe my report got boxed up when Mom went through her spring-cleaning frenzy.

My eyes widened as I stood in the middle of our basement, surrounded by mounds of boxes, and forgotten toys. My gaze landed on an ornate box with swirling patterns of vibrant colors covering every inch. I peeked under the lid and uncovered an album stuffed with pictures on top. My interest piqued, I lifted the album from the box and carried it upstairs.

As I settled onto the couch, I opened the album, my eyes glued to the first picture. It was of a lady, with a little girl on her lap -- their faces beaming at the camera. Was it a mother and a daughter, perhaps? I held the album closer to my face to study their features more. To my astonishment, the lady in the picture looked like Mom, except she was wearing weird, old-timey clothes. And, the little girl looked like me, except she was much chubbier.

Memories filled every page of the album. There were shots of birthdays and holidays from when the little girl was a baby until she was about my age. I traced my fingers around each photo, smiling at their happiness. I wondered who they were. Not only did they look similar, they felt familiar. I couldn't wait until Mom got back home so I could ask her.

Soon after that thought, Harmony and Hudson, who were sleeping beside me on the couch, bolted towards the kitchen. They knew Mom and Joey were back before the garage door even opened. In a frenzy, the dogs announced their arrival with authority and welcomed them home.

Lunch in hand, Mom set the pizza box on the counter and called for Dad. Joey plopped on the chair next to me at the table and tore into the box, snagging a slice of pepperoni and shoving it in his mouth.

"You must feel better," I mumbled under my breath. He looked at me and gave an open-mouthed smile, bits of chewed pizza coating his teeth. Disgusted, I grabbed my plate and moved to the counter barstool.

After listening to Mom tell Dad about Joey's ear infection and their trip to the store to pick up his medicine, I was waiting for an opportunity to steal Mom and show her what I discovered.

I walked to the couch and picked up the album I left lying on the pillow. When Mom glanced my way, I waved the book, signaling her to join me. As soon as she sat next to me, I shoved the album in her hands and turned to the first page. "Mom, who are they?" I pointed at the picture.

She gave a tender smile and placed her hand over her heart. "I haven't looked at these pictures in a long time," she said softly. "Don't you recognize them?"

I nodded my head. "This lady looks like you," I pointed to the little girl on the lady's lap. "And she looks kinda like me . . . but, how is that possible?" I asked puzzled. "She's bigger than me, and they are both wearing old-fashioned clothes."

Mom laughed, "The lady in the picture is your grandmother, Momo. And, that chubby little girl is me." As she turned to the next page, I realized how much sense that made. No wonder they felt familiar!

"Wow," I breathed in awe. "You're Momo's mini-me!" I exclaimed.

Mom chuckled and ruffled my hair. "And you're my mini-me!" she said lovingly.

I stared at her dumbfounded and must have looked funny as Mom covered her mouth and chortled. We stared at each other for a minute before dissolving in tear-inducing laughter.

"Don't look so offended, Lizbeth!" Mom laughed, wiping the tear that escaped. "I'm not . . . It's just that . . . you were a big girl!" I stammered. "Am I that chubby too?"

"No, sweetheart," she said, placing her hand on my arm. "I grew into myself, just like you will when you get older." She gave me a reassuring hug before leaving the couch. She placed the album on the counter by her purse. "We should show Momo these pictures when we see her tomorrow. She'll get a kick out of seeing these again."

I nodded my approval and thought more about what Mom had said about growing into myself. It made sense. Mom wasn't that chubby girl in the pictures anymore. That had to mean I wouldn't be chubby for too much longer myself—right?

5. Mean Kids

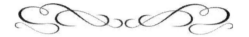

scanned the cafeteria for my two best friends. *T.G.I.F.* I started for our usual table, but when I found it full of the popular kids, I froze, swiveling my head to find friendly faces. Out the corner of my eye, I saw Hannah standing on top of the bench at a table in the far back, waving her hands in the air. Our friend Chelsea was next to her, laughing as she joined Hannah in their attempt to signal me amidst the sea of students.

With my lunch tray in hand, I strode towards them and faltered for a moment as I passed by Suzy. She was the only kid at her table, her eyes cast down as she morosely ate her sandwich. She looked so lonely. I wanted to ask her to join us but realized I would take the only seat available at our table, and there wouldn't be enough room for her.

As soon as I sat down, Hannah and Chelsea bombarded me with questions about the weekend.

"My dad got me and my cousin tickets to see Maximum Value this weekend!" Hannah squealed, clapping her hands. "Can you believe it?" she continued, bouncing in her seat.

"OMG, Hannah!" Chelsea exclaimed, grabbing Hannah's hand. "Get their autograph for me!" she pleaded. "I have to have it, pleaaaase."

I made the appropriate girlish response, smiling and encouraging Hannah to continue gushing about her favorite band, but my eyes and thoughts wandered, and their voices became a hum. I glanced over at Suzy. She was preparing her things and about to walk over to the garbage to throw out the remains of her lunch when another student blocked her. Suzy was now in front of mean girl territory -- Megan Selter's table.

"Where are you goin,' Fat Suzy?" questioned the girl, standing with crossed arms and blocking Suzy from going any farther. She stood there with a smug smile on her face when Suzy didn't respond.

"Hey, Suzy, fat doozy, your fat makes me woozy," cackled another of Megan's crew. The sting of the cruel words was like a punch in the face.

"Why are you walking? You should just roll to the garbage," Megan sneered as she rose from her seat. She strutted around the table and walked up to Suzy, jabbing a finger at her chest. "Listen up, you fat tub of lard," she said. "Don't you ever pass by our table again. You go around." She smiled, an evil glint in her eyes. "I don't want to throw up my lunch just seeing you roll by." Megan let her finger drop from Suzy's chest and stood to the side to let her pass.

With her head hanging, Suzy fled the cafeteria in tears. I looked around to the other tables, seeing if there were any witnesses to what just happened. To my dismay, people were carrying on, as if none the wiser. Did they see what happened and ignore it? Was there too much noise where they couldn't hear the disgusting and mean words thrown at Suzy?

I turned to Chelsea and Hannah, hoping they heard. My face fell as I realized there wasn't a break in their discussion about the concert this weekend. It appeared everyone ignored the situation -- ignored Suzy and the pain she must have felt.

As I sat staring at the empty table that Suzy left, I became mad. Mad that no one stepped in. Mad that no one scolded Megan and her mob of nasty friends, but most of all, mad at myself for doing nothing -- just like everyone else.

The rest of that day went by in a blur; my thoughts never straying far from Suzy. She had no one to stand up for her. Knowing that made me want to cry. At least I had Hannah and Chelsea. We had been close friends since kindergarten and always had each other's backs. If I were on the receiving end of some kid's mean remark, Hannah and Chelsea would swoop in and put a stop to it. Then they would spend an entire day coming up with silly things to do, anything to make me smile again and forget my pain.

I couldn't forget Suzy's pain. I had to be her support. I made a promise to myself that if I saw her being bullied again, I would say something. I would not sit and pretend that I didn't hear or see how mean those jerks acted.

~

By Sunday night, I was eager to go to school the next day. I hadn't thought of it Friday, but I should have had Hannah, Chelsea, join Suzy and me at her empty table. I would make certain that the three of us would sit with her tomorrow.

However, Monday came and went without Suzy. I figured she was sick and called in. Not that I blamed her.

Then, the whole week went by, and she was still missing. Towards the end of the week, I overheard a teacher speaking with the principal. Suzy went to live with her aunt in another town and would not be returning to Haven Hills Elementary.

The rumor around the school was just the opposite and was started by Megan and her puppet groupies. It spread like wildfire that Suzy was now living at a fat farm because she was too big to attend regular school.

My heart broke for Suzy as I wondered why she moved in with her aunt instead of staying with her parents. I thought about what I would have done had I been in Suzy's shoes. If I were in the same predicament, alone without best friends for assurance, I wouldn't want to come back to school either.

What would my day have looked like had Suzy been there and was being bullied again? Would I have made good on my promise by standing up to Megan and her mob? Could I have made things different for Suzy or any kid that got picked on?

6. The Worst Day

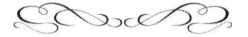

I was dreading going to school today. My usual sunny demeanor dampened at the thought I wouldn't have my two back-ups throughout the day. Hannah and Chelsea's homeroom had a field trip to an art museum today. It was so unfair! We'd had the same homeroom assignment since kindergarten, but this year, our final year at Haven, our streak ended. They said it was because of "over-crowded classrooms" or whatever nonsense. Mr. Harris, our principal, gave me that excuse when I barged into his office demanding answers for this year's placement at the start of the school year.

To make matters worse, Mom told me I had to take the bus this morning since she and Momo couldn't drive me. I stood on the sidewalk brooding and miserable when I felt the first splash of a cold raindrop land on my arm. *Are you kidding me?* I thought, lifting my head, and cursing the sky. The clouds darkened and swelled, threatening to burst with rain. I wiped the stray drop off my skin and prayed the bus would make it before the downpour. It didn't.

24

No one sat next to me on the bus. I figure they were afraid of getting wet since I was drenched. One kid dared to mention I should have worn a raincoat or grabbed an umbrella. I gave him a fierce look as I wrung the water from my hair, and he sank in his seat without another word.

I was mostly dry by lunch period. Almost jogging to the cafeteria, my plan was to arrive early enough to pick out an available table. I wasn't in the mood to search for people to sit with during lunch.

When I arrived, there was only a handful of students in line for food. Smiling to myself, I was happy with this one small break in this horrific day. Spotting an empty table in the back corner, I sprawled a few of my things across it, claiming it as my own. I opened my social studies book to a random page, hoping that if I buried my nose in it, then people wouldn't bother to join me.

About halfway through lunch, I heard someone clear her throat. I glanced up from my book to see Megan at my table, her fingers tapping an impatient rhythm on the hard surface. I panicked, my heart racing as I stared at her with wide, unblinking eyes. My fight-or-flight responses were at war with each other.

She seemed to enjoy my discomfort, turning to give her table a wide, wicked smile. Her friends laughed in encouragement. I shivered in disgust for the way she was enjoying the spotlight, reveling in the show she was putting on.

"Lizbeth," she started. "You know you can't sit here, right?" She cocked her head to the side like a dog, waiting for my response.

"Um . . . It was a free table," I retorted. "I'm not sitting at your table."

"You are obviously not sitting at my table!" she exclaimed, laughing at the thought. Her so-called friends cackled with her like a bunch of robots programmed to do everything she does.

She wiped a fake tear from her eye. "Oh, Lizbeth," she said. "You are quite the comedian." She stood and pointed to a table on the other side of the room. "That table over there is your new table!" she exclaimed. "That's where Suzy used to sit. And, since you're a fat loser like she was . . ." Her words hung there as she spun her hand, waving me on to finish her thought.

I sat there, flabbergasted. I couldn't believe this was happening. *It was already the worst day ever, and now this?* My mind spiraling, I looked back at Megan like a deer in headlights.

Her face scrunched in fury since I didn't respond the way she wanted me to. "Move to the fat table, Lizbeth! Now!" she spat, the veins at her temple pulsing. "Better yet . . . why don't you join the fat farm with Suzy?" She spun on her heels and marched back to her own table, her friends drowning in laughter at my expense.

I stood up and gathered my books. I looked at my tray of uneaten food and felt queasy. The voices of students melding with Megan's guffawing table and the smell of greasy fried food made me dizzy. I needed to get out of here. I wouldn't walk to the "fat table" and face even more humiliation. I was already ashamed of the tears streaming down my face. I didn't want to add to Megan's victory.

Despite a teacher's protest that I was leaving before lunch period was over, I walked straight to the nurse's office. I told the nurse that I was feeling nauseous and dizzy and would like to go home. She saw the tear tracks on my face and asked if there was anything else going on. I denied anything else but being sick.

I was lying on the cot with a damp towel over my eyes when I heard Momo's voice in the office adjoining the room I was in. She murmured to the nurse, asking how I was feeling and what her medical opinion was on this "sudden illness" I was experiencing.

I rolled my swollen eyes and sighed, knowing deep down my grandma could look straight to the truth. She had a knack for just knowing things. It made it impossible to get away with anything.

I sat up and groaned for good measure when the nurse entered the room with Momo trailing behind her. Although I was feeling horrible, I felt I needed to amp it up so I could milk it for a few days.

Momo's smug, all-knowing smile faded when she saw my expression. She replaced it with a concerned, fretful grimace. She rushed over and embraced me. "Oh, baby girl," she cooed. "Let's get you home and feeling better."

I must look worse than I feel if Momo was falling over herself to take care of me. Let's hope my acting skills would pay off. The thought of returning to school without a plan was enough to make me sick.

7. The Girl of My Dreams

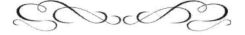

After crawling into bed, Momo tucked the blanket edges snuggly around my body. She planted a kiss on my forehead and asked me if I wanted some of her famous, "cure-all-ailments," chicken noodle soup. I loved her homemade soup, but with my stomach in knots, I felt I should skip eating. I shook my head and gave her a weak smile as my eyes drifted shut. She gave another tender kiss to my cheek and left, the door closing with a soft *snick*.

Waiting until I heard her footsteps fade, I sat upright in bed. Padding over to my bookshelf I swiped my favorite book, determined to get lost in a fantasy world. I wanted to turn off my thoughts for at least a little while.

After three chapters in, I nodded off in a fitful sleep. Every little noise woke me including the dogs barking, Perkins scratching my door, and Momo talking on the phone. I flopped in my bed like a fish out of water, just tossing and turning for what seemed like hours.

When Mom got home, she peeked into my room. I opened one eye when I heard her approach as she touched my forehead to check for fever.

"Hey there, Lizbeth," she whispered. "Are you feeling any better?"

I winced as she turned on the light near my bed. "Not at all," I moaned. I made a show of struggling to sit up, my arms shaking with the exertion.

On cue, Mom pushed me back down, her lips pursed in concern. "Just stay in bed, honey," she insisted. "Are you hungry at all? I can bring you up soup or something?"

My stomach rumbled as she mentioned food, just realizing that I had eaten very little of anything all day. "Can I have a bowl of cereal instead?" I asked, picturing the Cookie Crisp box in the pantry. I prayed that Joey hadn't eaten all my favorite cereal.

A short while later, Mom came in with the sugary cereal and a bowl of milk for me. "When you're done, just leave everything on your nightstand. I'll come by later to check on you." She pressed her lips on the side of my temple and squeezed my hand before leaving the room.

After devouring two servings of the cookie cereal, I clenched my stomach in pain. It felt as though there was a lead weight in there, bouncing against the walls of my tummy. The queasy feeling worsened, and I was afraid I would throw up. I darted to the bathroom when the throw-up feeling turned into a diarrhea explosion situation. I must have sat there on the toilet until I was empty and hollowed out.

Exhausted, I climbed back into bed and rubbed soothing little circles around my sore stomach. As I closed my eyes, I vowed never to eat Cookie Crisp cereal again.

BECOMING MISS IZZY

Throughout the night, I had the most vivid dreams.

In one, I was a massive balloon in the Thanksgiving Day Parade. Millions of people around the world saw my bloated body on display, tethered by a rope so I wouldn't fly away in the wind.

In another, I was at a summer birthday pool party, having no business wearing the newest two-piece swimsuit that was all the rage. I was embarrassed beyond words when I jumped in and emptied all the water from the pool. I pulled myself out and sobbed, my tears refilling the pool. I looked like a beached whale, all sprawled out on the deck.

Even my dream about the best holiday of the year was depressing. I was on a field trip with my homeroom at a ski resort right before Christmas. A group of students, all donned in their winter attire, had just returned from a sleigh ride. They scampered off, singing holiday tunes with glee as they made their way over to a gazebo to get cookies and hot chocolate. However, I was already there, looking like a huge abominable snowman as I devoured every cookie on the serving tray. The look of horror on everyone's face was clear, and I could not hide my shame. To make it worse, my classmates joined in song, voicing a new and twisted version of "Frosty the Snowman."

"Oh, naughty snowman, you're a jolly and fat soul. All of us you beat, you ate all our treats, now you really just should go. Oh, dear fat Lizbeth, why did you do that? Don't you know it's wrong; it didn't take you long; all that food has made you fat!"

Jolted awake, it surprised me to find my pillow damp. I must have been crying in reality at the same time as in my dreams. *No, not dreams*, I thought. *Nightmares.*

I turned my pillow over and lay back down, willing myself to fall back asleep and dream of pleasant things. It must have worked because my nightmares faded into something amazing.

As the dream began, I watched a beautiful, sun-kissed girl walk with confidence toward the welcoming doors of Ravenhurst Middle School. She was dressed like a young fashionista in a trendy outfit. Her hair was styled in the cutest way to frame her slender face. As I watched her every move, she felt familiar, like I knew her.

I admired her boldness, her fierce determination that showed in every step she made. When her hand reached for the door handle, she turned and waved a final goodbye to the silver-haired lady who had dropped her off at the curb. The girl and lady were smiling as they blew each other a kiss.

I recognized that silvery hair and loving face -- Momo! And, that captivating girl was me! It was as if my eyes were playing tricks on me. Unbelievably, the girl was me, but this girl was everything I was not—brimming with confidence, bubbly, striking, and not fat!

She was also kind and lent a compassionate ear to other kids feeling lost or out of place. This amazing girl didn't tolerate bullying. She stood up for those being picked on without fear of retaliation. Popular and outgoing, she got along with everyone.

When I woke in the morning, I felt a pang of longing deep inside me. I so wanted to be this new version of myself. It disappointed me when I sprinted to the mirror to see the same old, regular chubby me.

When Mom came in to check on me, she found me staring at my reflection, tears streaming down my face.

8. Facing the Truth

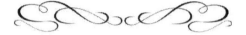

I sat on the edge of the top stair, peering between the posts on the handrail. Mom was trying to be discreet as she talked on the phone. Straining to hear, I assumed it was with Momo based on the tone of the conversation. Sighing, I wrapped an arm around my middle. My stomach felt raw yet angry with hunger. That's a feeling that Mom liked to call, "hangry." Even worse was the pain in my heart.

My thoughts drifted from one memory to another. *I remembered the time when Mom witnessed my despair in front of the mirror. She embraced me, cradling my head in the crook of her neck. She held me until my sobs subsided, the tear-stained spots drying on her shirt. I said nothing, even after she waited for me to answer her question. I was grateful for her comfort, but irritated that she had lied for so long.* I realized that all those times I questioned her about my weight, she looked right into my eyes and was still untruthful.

"Lizbeth!" she called, interrupting my thoughts. "Can you come down here, please?"

With a sense of dread, I descended the stairs and found Mom sitting at the dining room table, the phone resting near her. She wore a loving smile on her face as I approached, waving her hand towards the chair in a gesture to join her. As I sat, I looked around the room, straining my ears to hear if anyone else was home.

"Your dad took Joey to his baseball game," Mom said. "I was hoping we could talk . . . have a heart-to-heart." She reached over, placing my hand in hers.

"Okay . . ." I replied with hesitation, not sure where this would lead.

"Well, I talked to Momo this morning," she started. "She was concerned about you and called the school yesterday evening to ask the nurse more questions." She paused, letting her words hang there.

With a sinking feeling, I knew the jig was up. My act could never fool Momo. I wondered how she knew things. Nobody was ever that intuitive! And, because I made her worry, Mom was staring at me with concern, her eyes watering with unshed tears.

"What else happened yesterday, Lizbeth?" she gripped my hand tighter. "You know you can tell me anything."

Slipping my hand out of hers, I grew tired of this game. "You already know!" I exclaimed. "Why even ask me? I can't believe Momo just didn't leave it alone!" Pushing the chair back with the need to scream or cry, I wanted to run from the room. I was frozen in place.

Mom's eyes widened in surprise. "Honey, your grandmother was just worried and needed answers. We both did. Please, Lizbeth, just sit down and let's talk," she pleaded, keeping a calm demeanor.

Refusing to sit, I instead stood there with my hands planted on my hips. "Fine!" I fumed. "You want to know what happened?" My voice rose higher with each word I said. Mom nodded for me to continue.

"I'm the fattest girl in school!" I choked out. "Megan and her stupid friends ganged up on me . . . told me I should go to a table reserved for fatties"—my voice wavered as hot tears pricked my eyes. "She told me I should join a fat farm." The tears spilled over as I stood there, humiliated once again by reliving the torturous events of yesterday.

Mom rushed around the table, enveloping me in her arms as she joined me in crying. I pushed her away, needing to say more. I leveled her with an angry look. "And you, Mom! How could you lie all this time?"

I held her gaze in defiance as she opened her mouth to respond, but she couldn't formulate any words.

"Every. Single. Time. I asked you... you looked me in the face and lied!" I continued, punctuating my words.

She waited for me to finish hurling spiteful words at her before answering me. "You're right. You are absolutely entitled to feel angry."

Gaping at her, I was in shock that she admitted I was right.

"It's hard for me to explain, honey, but I'll try," she continued, holding her hand out for me to take. With hesitation, I took it.

She led me to the family room, where we sat on the couch. Perkins jumped on the cushion next to me and pawed at my leg, begging for attention. I stroked the top of his head between his down-like ears, awarding me with a vibrating purr of contentment. As he settled on my lap, Harmony and Hudson leaped on the couch, approaching me with slight trepidation. My hand held out welcoming them; I received doggy love as they both planted wet, sloppy kisses all over my face and nuzzled my neck. Mom and I laughed, breaking the tension between us. Animals are so forgiving and compassionate. They always know when I am upset and come to the rescue to make things better.

After the dogs calmed down and lay by my feet, Mom turned towards me. "It's not much of an excuse, Elizabeth," she started. "But I never answered you with complete honesty because I didn't want to hurt you, or have you doubt yourself." She paused, closing her eyes, and taking a deep breath, "I know what it's like being a bigger girl myself at your age. I hated what people said about me, but worst of all," she opened her eyes and met mine, pain etched on her features. "I hated myself."

I tore my gaze from hers, biting my lip. I couldn't stand to watch her pain mirror mine. I related to her thinking. I understood what it was like to observe your pretty skinny friends when meanwhile you stood out like a big fat Pillsbury Doughboy.

"I don't want you to hate yourself ever," Mom spoke. "You're a beautiful, smart, giving person that has so much to offer the world." She draped an arm around my shoulders, drawing me in to rest my head against hers. "I will do everything I can to make things better. We are a team and can work together so that you can be healthy and happy." She moved her head to seal a kiss on my cheek. "Does that sound like a plan? Do you forgive me?" she asked.

I looked into her adoring eyes and felt her love radiate around me. How could I not forgive her? I wasn't sure how she would fix it, fix me, but I realized I trusted her and that I wanted her guidance.

I never understood it until today, but one of Mom's sayings suddenly made sense, "Where there's a will, there's a way."

9. Going to Die

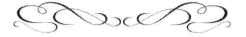

When I opened my eyes Monday morning, the smell of hot, doggy breath assaulted me. Harmony's head was lying on the pillow next to mine sound asleep. She must have crawled into bed with me in the night. I smiled, petting her side as her tail thumped the bed in a lazy wag. I glanced at the clock on my nightstand and jumped up in a panic, sending Harmony bounding out of the room. It was after 9:00 AM! No one woke me up for school!

I raced into the hallway, calling for Mom. I couldn't imagine anyone would leave me here home alone!

Mom peered up at me standing on the landing of the stairs and laughed at my frantic, disheveled state. "Don't worry, sweetie," she said. "No school for either of us today!"

I stood there confused, running a hand through my hair.

"Come on down. I made us some breakfast!" she called, walking into the kitchen.

I followed behind her and watched as she scooped eggs from the pan. When I chose my seat at the counter, she placed a glass of fresh-squeezed orange juice next to my plate. My breakfast looked so colorful! Scrambled eggs mixed with peppers and mushrooms with a side of blueberries and strawberries. I didn't remember the last time I'd eaten a breakfast like this. I didn't think I'd ever had a breakfast like this! My go-to was a bagel or Pop-Tart. If I were in a daring mood, I would snag cookies to eat on the ride to school.

With a little trepidation, I took a bite and surprised myself with how good it tasted. As I finished my meal, I asked, "Mom, what's going on?"

"I made a doctor's appointment for you this afternoon," she explained. "I figured we could spend time together. I know Momo wants to see you too."

It excited me to play hooky from school and spend time with Mom and Momo, but I was wary about having to go to the doctor. I already felt better after having my first heart-to-heart with Mom over the weekend.

"Why do I have to go to the doctor?" I asked. "I feel fine."

Mom leaned over the counter and plucked a stray blueberry from my plate to pop in her mouth. "Remember our deal about getting healthy and happy?" she asked with a grin. "Well, that starts with a trip to Dr. Adams to see where we're at. Plus, you'll need a physical anyway before you start middle school."

I tried to remember the last time I'd seen Dr. Adams. Joey was like his adopted son, considering how much time he spent with him.

I shrugged my shoulders in a matter-of-fact fashion. I could handle a visit to the doctor if it meant spending the entire day with Mom and Momo. It couldn't be that bad, right? Joey always seemed to bounce back whenever he went.

Mom clapped her hands in excitement, gaining the dogs' attention. "It's so nice outside today, how about we take Harmony and Hudson to the dog park?" she suggested, grabbing the leashes off the wall hook.

At the mention of "dog park," Harmony and Hudson jumped in unison, twirling around each other in glee and anticipation. We hadn't gone to the park for a long time, so this was a major treat for them!

Mom and I laughed at the dogs' silliness as she tried to contain them enough to hook their leashes on. "We can stop by Momo's for lunch afterward," she said, wrangling the dogs to the car.

Our time at the dog park was fun! Mom and I talked about the situation with Megan and her crew of evil bandits. We planned a way for me to avoid further humiliation. We laughed as we thought of things to say in response to their vile slander. Rather than stoop to their level of meanness, the plan we developed used the opposite tactics. We designed our plan to "kill them with kindness," so to speak. It was hard being mean to someone if you showered them with compliments. At least I hoped that was the case, but time would only tell.

The downside of this trip to the park was after walking one lap around the woodsy area, I was about ready to die of exhaustion. Maybe I wouldn't even make it to my doctor's appointment. I did not understand where dogs got so much energy, but I wished they would lend me some of theirs.

By the time we dropped the dogs off back home and went to grandma's, it was time for lunch. I was starving after all that exercise; my breakfast had worn off. My stomach rumbled as I dreamed of Momo's famous crispy fried chicken, a million times better than the Colonel's!

I opened the door and inhaled, seeking the aroma of the savory meal she prepared. I smelled nothing other than the musty floral pot-pourri she kept in a bowl on the foyer table.

"Is that you, my sweet Miss Izzy?" Momo called out from the kitchen.

I peeked around the corner, grinning when I saw her fuss at the dining room table. She was smoothing the cloth and adjusting a crooked candle in the candelabra that served as a centerpiece.

My eyes widened when she moved to the side of the table, giving me a full view of the spread, she put together with great TLC. There were glass bowls adorned with fresh flowers on each side of the candle centerpiece. The soft glow from the flames highlighted the crystal stemware as little shards of rainbows danced along the tablecloth.

"It's so beautiful, Momo!" I exclaimed as her eyes lit up with pride.

"I'm so glad you like it! After all, this is a special feast for my special girl," she said. "I hope you're hungry!" She waved at the chair, encouraging me to sit.

When she brought out the bowls of food, I tried not to let my disappointment show. I guess it would have been a feast if I enjoyed rabbit food. But as she beamed from ear to ear, describing how she cut every veggie for the massive salad she made, I realized I couldn't hurt her feelings. With as much enthusiasm as I could muster, I piled my plate and dug in.

Maybe it's because love surrounded me or because I was so famished after my trip to the park, but the food was tasty!

I admit—I felt special at the moment. Sitting at a beautifully decorated table with two of my most favorite people made me feel like a princess. Mom and I shared the highlights of everything we talked about with Momo, our time flying by with laughter and a stronger bond between the three of us.

As we prepared to leave, Momo wrapped me in a hug, planting a kiss on my forehead. "Good luck at the doctor, Miss Izzy," she said with a wink and then waved goodbye as we walked to the car.

It felt like we waited hours before Dr. Adams entered the exam room. And when he did, I was so anxious I couldn't wait for the visit to be over. Time seemed to stand still as I endured being weighed, measured, poked, and prodded. The doctor asked Mom all these questions about me as if I wasn't sitting right there.

After a full analysis, he labeled me as "overweight," which is just fancy talk for fat. He droned on about awareness of juvenile diabetes and heart disease. The importance of having a healthy diet was emphasized, along with exercise.

Mom's arms were full of pamphlets and guides on food and fun activities to "Get Kids Moving!" as the title proclaimed. Dr. Adams also provided her with information on a nutritionist and health coach should she need any guidance.

I sat there, half-amused, watching Mom try to absorb everything the doctor threw at her. Since she had a deer-caught-in-headlights look of puzzlement on her face, Dr. Adams turned his attention towards me. "We can count this visit as your middle school physical, but I'd like to see you again at the end of summer to see how things are going," he said with a smile, shaking my hand.

As we left the office, that voice in my head chattered. I realized I should have listened when Dr. Adams was talking about diseases caused by fat. *Did he say I have diabetes and heart disease? Or was it a warning, a disaster waiting to happen?* I felt overwhelmed, scared that I wouldn't be able to turn things around. I promised Mom we would work as a team, but—what if I got sick and died? The worry gauge in my head was now on high alert.

As much as Mom tried to be upbeat on the ride home, I was not in the mood. I hated to ruin what started as an amazing day, but I stayed silent, retreating deep in my thoughts as my worries threatened to drown me in a tide of despair.

After we pulled into the garage, Mom twisted in her seat to face me. "What's on your mind?" she inquired, resting her hand on mine.

I glanced at her, blowing out the deep breath trapped inside me. "It's all so confusing, Mom. I am worried and scared. Should I be?" The words tumbled out as I spilled my worried thoughts. "Am I sick? Do I have diabetes? Will I die?" I choked on that last question, terrified of her answer.

Before I could ask anything else, she gripped my hand and spoke with determination. "I hear you, and I am with you, so don't be afraid. You do not have diabetes, and you will not die." She paused, waiting for her words to sink in.

I gave a meek nod before she continued.

"We will take this one day at a time. We will go slow. Everything will not change overnight." She smiled, and her voice grew softer. "I want you to share how you are feeling every step of the way and ask me questions. I promise I will explain things to you and answer all your questions."

Mom's pep talk worked. It relieved me to find out I wasn't dying of diabetes or some other awful fatty disease! However, I couldn't help but wonder what all this change would look like. *Do I have it in me to do it?*

Mom moved her hand to my face, lifting my chin to look her in the eyes, which were glowing with a purpose. "Deal?" she asked me.

I grinned at her resolve, nodding my head in approval. "Deal," I said.

We walked into the kitchen and discovered a note on the counter. Mom picked up the letter and read it, a smile spreading across her face.

"What's it say?" I asked with curiosity, trying to peer at the note in her hands.

She set the paper down, looking at me. "Want to continue our girl's day out?"

I raised my eyebrows in response. Didn't she have to make dinner for Dad and Joey? I glanced around the room and realized most of the lights were off, signaling we had an empty house. "Where's Dad and Joey?" I asked perplexed.

"The note was from your dad. He has a golf thing with his buddies, and your brother is at a sleep-over," she replied, almost bouncing with delight. "Let's grab Momo and continue our girls-only day! We can go out to dinner, your pick! Whatever your heart desires!"

Her enthusiasm was contagious as we clasped hands and danced in a little circle. Laughing, I shouted my approval as she grabbed the phone to call Momo.

At my favorite restaurant, Chipper's Roadhouse, the three of us talked about the upcoming summer while we pigged out on some good ole' fashioned country comfort food. With a twinge of agony, I realized I wouldn't get to eat like this much longer. I would have to learn to enjoy rabbit food from now on if that was even possible.

"Do you think this will be hard to do? Stop eating bad foods, even if they are my favorite?" I asked them, pausing before I added, "Or could we at least make it fun?" I wasn't even sure how that would be achievable.

Mom looked at Momo, who gave a nod of encouragement. "I think that will depend on what you want it to be, honey," she responded with a smile. "I say we make this an adventure!"

My grandma clapped, agreeing with this sentiment.

"An adventure!" I exclaimed. Being an avid reader, I loved adventures! They didn't always run as planned or without bumps in the road. But, being on the adventure would be worth it. "When will our adventure start?" I asked.

Mom looked up, the wheels turning as she devised a plan. "Well, we have about five weeks before school is out for summer," she started. "We use that time to plan and get ready by doing little things each day and focusing on making the end of elementary school special. Those small things we do each day will get us ready for a big summer adventure," she declared. "How does that sound?"

I nodded, feeling a little more confident. With Mom and Momo with me every step of the way, how could it go wrong? I trusted them to make this work, and to my surprise, I recognized I believed in myself.

10. Enjoying the Ride

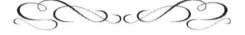

F*inally! It's summer. Almost three whole months doing things I want to do!*

The final bell rang, and kids everywhere shouted in glee and danced out of the main doors of Haven Hills Elementary School. It was my last year in this school, and the thought of never seeing Mr. Landry again filled me with a sadness that sunk like a lead weight in my chest. He was my favorite teacher, helping me when things got rough with Megan and her snotty friends. It was hard to believe all that changed in the last five weeks, and now I had a summer adventure to look forward to.

I sat on the smooth stone steps at the entrance of Haven Hills as I waited for Momo to arrive. I turned my face to the sky and closed my eyes as the early summer sun warmed me. I wondered what my first day of sixth grade would look like. Most of the friends I made at Haven Hills would go to the new middle school one town over. But because of what my mom called "boundary lines," I would go to the one located three blocks from

45

our house, Ravenhurst Middle School. Would the kids be nice there? Would I make new friends?

I moved my hand to my chest, trying to rub the little twinge of pain that settled there. I would miss my friends, Chelsea, and Hannah. The three of us had known each other since kindergarten. No one ever picked on me and called me mean names when they were around. They gave me the courage to stand up to Megan and other bullies.

I wondered how things might have turned out that day Megan took over my table if Chelsea and Hannah hadn't been on a field trip. I might not have gone home sick. Mom and I may not have had our first heart-to-heart. The trip to see Dr. Adams might not have happened when it did. There wouldn't be a plan to stand up to mean kids. I might not have planned a summer adventure with Mom.

My eyes fluttered open as a car horn brought me back to the present. I squinted my eyes as they adjusted to the bright sunshine, and I saw Momo waving from her car window.

"C'mon, Miss Izzy!" she shouted. "Let's not waste a single moment of this summer!"

Shaking off my worried thoughts, I grabbed my bag and sprinted down the steps towards my grandma's car, a huge smile consuming my face. Before reaching the handle of the car door, I looked back at Haven Hills and whispered a silent goodbye.

"Looks like something was on your mind back there, Miss Izzy," Momo commented. "Want to talk about it?"

I twisted in my seat for a more comfortable position and looked at my grandma's face. She was one of my most favorite people in the world. I stared at the silvery gray hairs framing her face and noticed several lines, wrinkles, and creases that appeared there. Momo was old. I never wanted to lose her. I already was about to lose having my two best friends at school with me.

As Momo looked over, I stuffed that worry in the back of my head to deal with later. "Nothing," I said in response, "Just glad it's summer!" I gave Momo my "million-dollar smile," as she liked to call it.

"I'm glad too," she replied, smiling in kind, and squeezing my hand with her free one. "We can talk about it later," she said knowingly.

How does she do that?

A mix of emotions assaulted me as we pulled away from the curb -- excitement, melancholy, anticipation, and relief.

I wished I was more like Momo. She had a way of just knowing things, but even though I lacked her intuitiveness, I still felt I was on the brink of something big. A feeling inside me and that voice seemed to know this would not be just any old summer. I could already hear my grandma's voice inside me, "It's time for your summer adventure, Miss Izzy. It will be one you will not forget. Enjoy the ride!"

PART II

ADVENTURE AND TRANSFORMATION

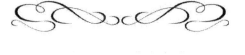

---

11. My Journey Through Hurt

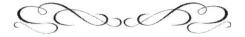

With my days at Haven Hills Elementary behind me and summer break laid out before me, Mom wasted no time to get our adventure started.

Not knowing what to expect, I found myself filled with doubt and worry. *Am I prepared to make all the changes everyone expected me to?*

Mom did her best to keep me positive, but I think she realized some of her efforts were in vain. One morning I found her fiddling with the stack of pamphlets and brochures Dr. Adams had given her. Her brow furrowed while she tapped one paper with her fingers until she finally gave in and made a call to Dr. Sue, the health coach recommended to us.

After her talk with the health coach, it appeared Mom gained the confidence she needed to kick things in gear. She bustled around the kitchen, humming a little tune while she prepared breakfast.

Mornings no longer included sugary cereal and chocolate milk. Healthier options replaced my breakfast of choice. Scrambled egg whites with cheese, sautéed colorful veggies, and turkey sausage were one option. Or, healthy "cereal" (as Mom would call it) was another—oatmeal made with milk and topped with an assortment of bright berries and crushed walnuts. Surprisingly, I realized I preferred both of these healthy options over my usual bowl of chocolaty sweetness.

While not letting on I enjoyed Mom's homemade breakfasts, not everyone was happy. Joey would throw a little tantrum, threatening to starve himself if he couldn't have what he wanted. Mom would cross her arms, unmoved by his outbursts. She looked to my dad for support, but he would just shrug his shoulders. Although he didn't openly complain, I could tell my father missed some of his favorite "unhealthy" foods.

As a compromise to the boys, Mom agreed to save one day on the weekend when we could have whatever we wanted to eat. The catch? One meal only. It was something to look forward to, so despite how my father and brother felt, I was fine with it.

Mom and I also took Harmony and Hudson on walks and trips to the dog park, much to their delight. They learned pretty quickly this was a daily routine.

Before summer, I would come home from school and beeline it to the fridge or cabinet in a desperate search for a snack to carry me through until dinner. Both dogs would eye me as I parked on the couch, chowing down while watching cartoons. And when they realized I wasn't giving up a morsel of food, they fell asleep by my feet.

Now? It was like the dogs had an internal clock and knew when it was time to head out. They could barely contain their excitement, their bodies wriggling and bumping into me while I struggled to walk across the kitchen to grab their leashes off the wall hook. Mom and I would laugh together every morning, amused by their eagerness. And because their enthusiasm was so contagious, I looked forward to our daily stroll around the neighborhood and frolicking in the park afterward.

Besides healthier eating and exercising with the dogs, Mom assigned another task; journaling. This time I complained. School was out, and it was summer for goodness' sake! I did not want to write every day like it was homework!

Mom, being ever-patient, assured me she would not grade or judge my journal entries. She said a journal was like a diary and would be for my eyes only unless I wanted to share what I had written with her. I could put all my thoughts, feelings, wishes, and worries on paper however I wanted. And, if I needed to reflect on something later on, I could refer back to my journal. She mentioned this might be "freeing" for me to express myself in this way.

As reluctant as I was to the journaling, it ended up being how Mom said it would be—freeing. And it often was the answer to my nagging thoughts. That "intuitive" voice in my head seemed to quiet down when I put my thoughts on paper.

Re-reading some of my entries over the last couple weeks revealed some interesting clues to what had been bothering me. I wrote about that unrelenting "sick" feeling that occurred in the pit of my stomach now and then. I would feel fine one moment, and the next a weird tightening sensation would spring up out of nowhere. Or, so it seemed.

It wasn't one of those, "I'm going to puke my guts out" or "I'm going to poop my pants" kind of sick feelings. However, it was still a queasy, fluttery feeling. Thankfully, I had the foresight to make a list in my journal whenever these ill feelings occurred. These proved to be telling.

#1 I'm nervous about middle school . . . Will Megan be there? Will she continue to harass me?

#2 I'm sad that I might never get to eat sugar again . . . or pizza.

#3 I think Mom and Dad are fighting more. Is it my fault?

#4 Middle school again—will new kids like me? Am I smart enough? Will I get good grades?

#5 Momo's old—will she die soon? I hate thinking about that happening.

#6 What if I hate the new me? Will I even lose any weight? Will I disappoint my family?

I found the connection and realized that had I not kept a journal; I might not have discovered my problem. Mom and Momo were right after all, I worried too much. Mr. Landry's talk about that seed we planted in science class came rushing back. All my worrying was making me hurt. Keeping everything buried inside, without expressing my emotions, was making me sick and scared.

Making this discovery, I was proud of myself. Now I knew I shouldn't bottle my feelings. I wanted to express myself even more. I found markers and decorated every inch of my journal cover with bright-colored patterns and doodles. I knew I would use this coveted book all throughout my summer adventure, and I couldn't be happier!

12. Sweet Without Sugar

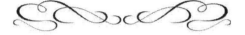

After a couple of weeks eating healthier meals, I came downstairs one morning expecting to see the oatmeal or eggs waiting for me. Instead, I saw Mom fanning paper across the kitchen island, a smile spread across her face.

"What's going on?" I asked, confused while stepping closer to see what the papers contained.

Mom clapped her hands together with an authoritative snap, directing my gaze away from the sheets on the counter. She grinned as I met her eyes. "We will play a little game!"

Before I could ask, she opened cabinet drawers and the door to the pantry, revealing the cans and boxes of food stacked on the shelves. I reached for one paper and read the title, "Curbing Sugar: Let the Hunt Begin!" Below that, there was a long list of names, most of which I couldn't even pronounce.

When Mom turned to face me, I shook the paper in her direction, questioning this "game."

"That, my dear Lizbeth," she said, referencing the list in my hands, "is a list of all the names for different sugars found in food."

She plucked the box of Cookie Crisp cereal from the pantry shelf and flipped it over to show the nutrition label. "Here are the ingredients," she pointed. "Compare that to the list on that paper. For example, dextrose, barley syrup, and the obvious one -- sugar."

She walked around the island and held up another piece of paper labeled "Dump." Beckoning me with her finger, she motioned for me to place the sugary cereal next to the paper. "This is the 'Dump' pile. Any foods you find that contain just one ingredient found on the 'Curbing Sugar' list will go in this pile."

I glanced at the remaining paper on the counter and read its title, "Keep." I faced Mom with uncertainty after peering inside the pantry. Was anything even going to land in the 'Keep' pile?

"We can do it!" she said. "And if we end up with a small 'Keep' pile, we'll just have to go shopping. It'll be fun!" Mom grabbed my hand, spinning me in a small circle as I laughed at her insistence.

I took her challenge to ditch the junk food-filled pantry and cabinets as just another challenge on this adventure. I'd already known there would be obstacles and difficulties on the journey. However, my brother did not share the same thought.

By the time Joey dragged himself from the bed and wandered into the kitchen, Mom and I had a hefty "Dump" pile going. He froze mid-step and rubbed the sleep from his eyes—that, or he had to assure himself that he was awake and not having a nightmare.

When reality sank in, his eyes bugged out like a comic character in disbelief as he witnessed us taking items from the "Dump" pile and throwing them in the trash.

"What are you doing?" he exclaimed in horror, sprinting across the room to rescue a package we'd thrown away. "Those chocolate sandwich cookies are my favorite!"

Undeterred, Mom snatched the cookies from his hands and tossed them back in the garbage. "We are having a scavenger hunt and must get rid of all the foods that are no good," she said, then softly added, "Would you like to help?"

"No good?" he wailed. "No good? Those cookies aren't just good, they're amazing!" he emphasized, stamping his foot like a toddler about to throw a tantrum.

I chuckled, unable to suppress my amusement at his theatrics. He glared at me, "You!" he pointed at me in an accusing manner. "You're helping her throw out all our good stuff?"

When I shrugged and gave him a "What are you gonna do?" look, he spun around. Then he did the unthinkable. He acted like a bratty little two-year-old throwing the biggest fit I'd ever seen. He dramatically flung himself on the floor, pounding his fists against the tile. His face turned a reddish purple from the effort he was making to cry.

"Joseph Ethan Tanlin!" Mom shouted, fed up. "Stop that right now!"

My brother stopped screaming and flailing his arms in that instant. A few more tears escaped as he lay there, his chest heaving as he tried to control his breathing.

Mom bent down, offering a hand to help him stand. "I know this is hard," she consoled. "And I know you don't see it now, but this will be good for all of us."

She wrapped him in a hug and rubbed soothing circles along his back to calm him.

"I think you would be amazing at this game," she suggested, trying to draw his interest.

My brother peeked around Mom for a better look at the piles stacked on the counter. Then he shifted his eyes to the garbage containing his beloved sandwich cookies.

"I don't see how," he mumbled. "What's in it for me? Besides throwing away everything I like?"

I could see the wheels turning in Mom's mind. She was attempting to come up with a way to keep Joey engaged. I stood there fiddling with the edge of the box I was holding while I waited for her response.

"Well, whoever wins at being the best sugar detective will get a prize," she paused for effect, "A twenty-five-dollar item of your choice on our next trip to the store." Joey and I both gaped at her, excited at this turn of events. "Non-food item! The prize excludes food," she added.

Now that there was a prize on the line, my brother seemed agreeable. "What do I have to do?" he asked.

Mom smiled and winked in my direction, happy that everyone was on board.

"Your mission, if you choose to accept it," she said, "is to read a label and see how many sugars you can find." She showed him the list outlined on the paper. "The challenge will be that once you find the sugar, you must be willing to 'curb' it."

I held up the "Dump" sign over my head so he could see it better.

Mom continued, "We'll keep track of how many we find. Agree to add any item with over one sugar on the label to the trashcan."

My brother nodded, "And if I find the most sugars, I can pick out whatever I want for twenty-five dollars?" he asked, smiling, no doubt thinking of a video game to add to his collection.

After Mom agreed, Joey grabbed the carton of Pop-Tarts from the cabinet, saying, "Let's get this started." He examined the ingredients and announced the treats had cane sugar, honey, and corn syrup. He tallied his score, kissed the box three times, one for each sugar, and dunked it in the trash like a pro-basketball player.

The three of us laughed at his silliness. Despite the rough start, we ended up having a lot of fun playing sugar detectives. I wasn't even jealous that Joey won. Mom was so proud we all worked together that she treated me to a mani-pedi while my brother scavenged the toy store with his prize money.

The next week without sugar was brutal. Joey was cranky, even more than his usual self. I had plenty of headaches and complained about it often. Momo used to say we were the "sweetest little thangs," but that week—we were far from it!

When I asked Mom why everyone was being so cranky and mean, she stated we were going through withdrawal. Because the body is so sensitive to sugar, the sugar acts like a drug and becomes addictive. When you go without it, your body detoxes— that means it goes through a process to get rid of poisons and chemicals in foods, like sugar—and the side effects are the ugly parts we have to get through.

However, after we made it through those ugly parts, things got much better. I felt great and had so much more energy! Even Joey acted like a different person. He seemed calmer and had fewer meltdowns. He was nice most of the time! Maybe we can be sweet—even without the sugar.

13. Healthy Shopping and Cooking

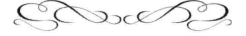

After a couple of weeks of "curbing" sugar, Mom asked me if I wanted to join her on a trip to Winn-Dixie to replenish our healthy stock. I was a little reluctant to go—after all, the sample booths were the best part of shopping there.

When she noticed my hesitation, Mom grabbed the list from the fridge door and handed it to me. "It'll be okay," she said, smiling, and nodding at the paper in my hands. "We'll resist temptation together because we have an attack plan."

As we made our way to the store, she talked about setting goals and making this trip another challenge: a game to beat. She was speaking animatedly, gesturing with her fingers to make her point. I sat silently, an amused smile on my face as I watched her flailing hands "speaking" a mile a minute.

"So?" she asked, her hands finally resting on the steering wheel. "What do you think?"

"Um..." I paused in an attempt to remember what she said, "Sure?" I couldn't admit that I was paying more attention to her floundering than her voice, but since I answered her with a question, she already knew. Momo's intuitiveness must be hereditary.

Rather than scold me, she repeated everything, although with less animation and gusto. Our plan was to shop the outer aisles first, loading up on fresh veggies, fruit, meat, and dairy before searching the boxed and canned food aisles. Our goal was to find at least two or three new foods to bring home with us. That way, we could experiment and not have to eat the same thing all the time. Like Momo would say, "Variety is the spice of life!"

We had a great time picking out our meals for the week. Mom mentioned I could be her mini-chef, and when I had enough training, we could compete to win my father and brother's favor. I laughed when she mentioned that. I didn't think we could ever persuade Joey to eat veggies. We already had to sneak healthier treats in his lunch bag and pretend that he got away with eating something bad for him. It was a minor victory when we noticed him adding the snack to the grocery list the next day.

The first-time broccoli made its debut at our dinner table; I thought my brother would throw his plate across the room. "I will not eat these green tree things!" he protested. "Veggies make me gag."

It wasn't until I asked if I could eat his roasted broccoli that he agreed to try it. He took the tiniest bite, a little green spore on his fork when his eyes went wide with amazement. He didn't gag one bit but nearly choked from the way he was shoveling the vegetable into his mouth. That ended up being a win!

Joey did not respond to every new dish as he did with his introduction to broccoli. There were meals in that first month I vowed never to make again. I played a big part not only in shopping for healthy foods but also in the meal planning and preparation. So, it thrilled me when Mom asked if I wanted to prepare a special meal for Momo's sixty-fifth birthday.

"Why don't you give your grandma a call and see what she wants?" Mom asked as she grabbed the phone from the dock and handed it over to me. "She'll be here early this evening, around four o'clock."

I smiled while dialing her number, thinking of the many unique and exciting meals I'd learned to make so far. I was excited to show off my new culinary skills.

"Well, hello there, Miss Izzy!" Momo greeted me. "Couldn't wait to wish your grandma a happy birthday?" she chuckled.

I couldn't help laughing in response. "How did you know it was me, Momo? You don't even have caller ID!"

In a serious voice, she replied, "I know everything."

Puzzled, I had to shake my head to get my thoughts in order. *How does she do that?*

"I was calling to see what you wanted for your birthday dinner tonight. Something special and homemade is what I am planning," I said with pride as I caught Mom's eye and winked. She gave me a silent thumbs-up before she bustled around the kitchen, wiping down the counters with disinfectant.

"Meatloaf!" Momo exclaimed. She was giddy with excitement. "I've wanted a delicious, juicy meatloaf for some time now. That will be perfect!"

Meatloaf? She has to be kidding. Who wants meatloaf for their birthday? My ideas for exotic cuisine deflated as I thought of her suggestion.

61

BECOMING MISS IZZY

Unable to talk her out of her choice of protein, I was still free to make whatever sides I thought would go best with it. It was a challenge to come up with a way to make an ordinary meatloaf an extraordinary one, but I was eager to try. I imagined I was on one of the kid's cooking shows, competing for the prized title of chef champion. I decided on making individual loaves, instead of the traditional meat-filled football. And, instead of using a packet of dry seasoning, I used fresh herbs from the garden that Mom and I started when summer began. For the sides: creamy mashed potatoes and garlic-roasted green beans.

Just before Momo arrived, I admired the feast I prepared. It reminded me of when my grandma went all out for our girl's day brunch with her table decorated to perfection and the massive rabbit-loving salad.

Joey strode in the kitchen, inhaling a deep breath through his nostrils before turning with a smile. "It smells so good, Lizbeth! I'm excited to eat whatever you made; even if it's veggies!" He laughed in disbelief at his own words. "I mean, if it smells that amazing, it can't taste that bad, right?"

When we sat at the table and devoured the meal I'd made with love, Momo shifted in her seat to look me straight in the eye. She had a warm smile spread across her face, her eyes glistening with unshed tears.

"You did an outstanding job, Miss Izzy. Everything tasted so wonderful!" she said. Then she wrapped me in a hug and whispered in my ear, "I think the only thing I love more than this meatloaf is the cook."

14. Fitness Fun

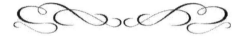

The next morning, two wiggling, enthusiastic dogs greeted me as I walked into the kitchen. I had slept in a little later than normal, and it was apparent I messed with their daily routine. Harmony kept nudging me with her nose, attempting to make me walk faster. Hudson ran in circles around me, darting in between my legs while giving an impatient, muffled bark.

"What's with you two?" I chuckled, pushing Harmony's cold, wet snout from my leg. "You'll get your walk!"

As soon as I uttered that magical word, "walk," Hudson charged into the kitchen and swiped the leash with his teeth from Mom's hand. She stood there, bewildered by his behavior. When he trotted over and dropped the leash by my feet with a loud bark, we burst into tear-inducing laughter.

"Let's not keep them waiting for a second longer!" Mom said, wiping her eyes.

We somehow wrangled the dogs long enough to attach their leashes and headed outside. I was grateful I had Harmony for this walk as she was much calmer than Hudson. A good distance ahead of me, it seemed Hudson was taking Mom for a walk instead of the other way around. She was almost sprinting to keep up with him!

She turned her head and shouted over her shoulder for me to pick up the pace. "C'mon, Lizbeth! Keep up with us!"

Harmony and I exchanged a wary look. Neither one of us wanted to run and keep up. We were quite happy with a leisurely stroll, but I realized Mom would continue to shout, creating a scene with Hudson's incessant barking. So, despite my unwillingness to exercise more than I had to, I jogged over and joined them.

As soon as we neared them, they took off again, keeping Harmony and me at a constant fast pace. I looked down at her to see if she was panting as hard as I was. To my disappointment, she was the picture of happiness with her mouth open wide in a doggy smile, her tongue lolling out the side.

"You traitor," I mumbled, my breath ragged. Harmony responded by licking my hand as if in encouragement.

I kept up the grueling pace for a while longer. I thought my legs would collapse under me. "Mom!" I gasped trying to yell. My lungs felt like they were on fire and about to explode. "I need a break!"

I was running, more like a shuffle since my legs felt like lead weights. Mom glanced back at me and paused, jogging in place.

"You can do it!" she exclaimed unconcerned. "Just make it to the park, and we can take a break there." She didn't even sound out of breath! I didn't know how I did it, but I gathered what little energy I had left and ran the rest of the way to our destination.

Over the next few weeks, I hit my stride on these daily walks. I even grabbed Hudson's leash and let Mom struggle with Harmony. Although we ended up having a good time with the dogs at the park, it became boring doing the same old thing every day.

When we started our walk one morning, I asked Mom if we could stick to only going through the neighborhood.

"You don't want to go to the park?" she responded, a surprised look on her face.

I shook my head, feeling a little guilty. I knew both dogs loved romping around and chasing each other with their big goofy, carefree canine smiles. "I wanted to know if we could do other things instead. It's getting kinda boring," I admitted, averting my eyes from Hudson and Harmony. I would hate to see their sad puppy-eyed looks of disappointment directed at me.

"Hmm . . ." she murmured, contemplating. "What do you have in mind?"

A ton of ideas popped into my mind as I spoke, "We could go to the beach and swim. Or the amusement park and zoo. Maybe I can try roller-skating. Or bowling!" I grew more excited with each suggestion.

Mom looked at me in disbelief although I could hardly blame her. Last summer, if someone had even suggested doing any of those activities, I would have whined and complained nonstop. I'd been content sitting around the house and doing as little as possible.

After a moment, she shook her head as if waving off her surprise and broke into a grin. "Those are wonderful ideas, Lizzy! We can plan our fitness activities like our shopping and meal planning for the week. What do you want to do first?"

"Hmm," I murmured, mimicking her earlier contemplation. I thought of soft, pliant white sand and the soothing sound of waves rippling along the shore as the warm summer sun caressed my face. "Definitely, the beach! Although." I paused, remembering a vital piece was missing, "I don't have a swimsuit."

Mom clapped her hands together, a sure sign of a plan in place. "Let's go shopping!" she said. "I could use a new one myself!"

Later that afternoon, I was standing in the store dressing room, staring at my image in the mirror and shocked by the reflection I saw. I looked good in the two-piece tankini bathing suit I was trying on. I smiled with pride, my eyes glistening, as I realized I wasn't ashamed for once in how I looked. Just two months into my summer adventure, I had lost sixteen pounds. I would have never guessed that fitness would be as much fun as it was, but this summer just continued to surprise me.

15. Healthy Around Food Junkies

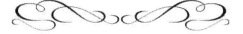

With Mom and Momo's support, my summer adventure was smooth sailing. It was easy making the right decisions being around them. But when an opportunity came up for a week-long trip without my family guiding me along, I was nervous I wouldn't have the strength to avoid temptation.

I was so proud of myself. I was able to deflect bad habits at a family event a couple of weeks ago at my cousin's birthday party. Even my Aunt Dee noticed the changes.

"Why Lizbeth!" she exclaimed, holding me at arm's length to get a better look at me. "It looks as though you're finally growing into yourself! You must have grown three to four inches! You're slimming down nicely!"

I cringed under her scrutiny but kept a smile plastered on my face. "Thank you," I replied politely, glancing over to find Momo glaring at Aunt Dee, a frown thinning her lips.

Momo sauntered to us and threw an arm over my shoulder. "Nice of you to notice," she snapped at my aunt. "My Miss Izzy sure is one beautiful young lady!" She softened her stance, planting a kiss on the top of my head.

When it had come time for cake, I accepted a small slice but declined the ice cream that was melting in a sugary pool from the heat. I ate slowly, savoring each bite. These kinds of treats had become rare, so I wanted to enjoy every moment.

With plenty left over, Aunt Dee called out for seconds. Before this summer, I would have been the first in line for more cake. My aunt looked surprised when I turned down her offer. Mom had flashed me a thumbs-up while Momo winked at me, proud of my determination.

That was all molehills compared to the mountain before me. Each day that took me closer to my week-long trip, I grew more and more anxious.

I met Rachel Collins during one of our roller-skating outings a few weeks ago. We became fast friends, laughing together as we raced around the rink and competing to see who the best skater was. Our mothers got along too, and we made plans to meet up several times a week doing different activities.

Rachel and her family moved to our town a few months earlier, and I was beyond excited to learn she would attend the same middle school as me in the fall. During one of our sleepovers, she invited me on a camping trip her family took every year.

It thrilled me, but despite our get-togethers, Rachel and her family didn't know I was on a healthier food plan. How was I going to keep that a secret during this trip? It would embarrass me if they knew.

People don't eat healthy on camping trips! Even though the thought of eating my way through a week of carb-filled comfort foods brought a twinge of joy to my heart, I didn't want to spoil all the progress I'd made. I was drooling just picturing a fluffy, fat marshmallow roasting over the campfire. The gooey sugar blob sandwiched between layers of chocolate and graham crackers— I couldn't turn that down! Wouldn't it be rude if I said no? I didn't want to ruin their family fun if I wasn't joining in.

Conflicted, I told Mom that I wasn't going.

"What?" she asked dumbfounded. "Why don't you want to go?"

I explained how I felt I wouldn't be able to say no when presented with temptation and that I would either ruin everything I was working towards or disappoint my friend.

"Don't be silly, you're stronger than you think," she said. "I'll just let Rachel's mom know you have certain dietary needs."

"No!" I shouted in horror. "Please, Mom, that's so embarrassing. Please, please, don't say that." I pleaded; my eyes welling with tears. I didn't want to lose Rachel as a friend because of a food downfall.

Mom reached for my hand, giving it a squeeze. "Okay, let's figure this out," she said. "You can't escape being around other people eating junk. Worse, you don't have to feel ashamed of the way you are eating," she stressed, moving around me to envelop me in a comforting hug. "You don't have to apologize if you feel the need to turn down something you don't want to eat. I have faith in you, Lizbeth."

Mom's words encouraged me. The camping trip was back on.

Later I realized I had nothing to fear when I overheard a conversation between both mothers. Because Rachel had diet restrictions for allergies, she couldn't eat a lot of preserved junk food either.

Having that knowledge, we all went on a shopping spree to find some healthy snacks for our trip. What a relief it was to find a friend who followed a similar diet.

I thought about Mom's words of wisdom, about being unashamed about how I was now eating or about turning down tempting offers. Had someone offered me roasted broccoli or a cup of fruit salad a few months ago, would it have been difficult for me to respond with a polite, "No, thank you"? Probably not. This was no different. In the future, if someone offered me something that I didn't want to eat, I could politely turn it down guilt-free.

16. Keeping This Secret Forever

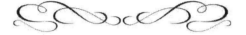

When the Collins family dropped me off at home after our camping trip, I sprinted for the door, eager to tell Mom all about it. I was expecting Harmony and Hudson to greet me with their barks and slobbery kisses as soon as I stepped through the threshold, but I heard complete silence. I was so disappointed.

I walked down the foyer and peeked around the corner into the kitchen. Nothing. "Hello?" I tentatively called. "Anybody home?"

I heard a muffled voice in response. With my heart hammering in my chest, I sought the noise with caution. Scared that something happened to my family, I crept along the wall towards the patio door. The screen door flew open and taken aback; I let out a panicked scream.

My dad filled the frame; his eyes widened in surprise at my reaction. Just as he was about to ask if I was okay, I busted out in laughter. "Sorry, Dad!" I chuckled. "You scared me!"

While berating me about almost causing him a heart attack, he gave me a huge bear hug, lifting me off my feet. It was something I hadn't felt in a while.

"Where is everyone?" I asked, looking around the empty room.

"Your Mom and Joey took the dogs to the park," he replied. "How was your trip? Did you have a good time?"

Before I could respond, he cocked his head as if puzzled, staring at me. "Look at you," he drifted off, talking more to himself than to me. "It's like you've changed right before my eyes!"

Deciding to ignore his comment, I launched into the events of the trip. "I had so much fun, Dad! Rachel is my new best friend. We have so much in common! We went swimming, hiking, and fishing almost every day. I even learned how to paddle a kayak! We caught fish for dinner, but I didn't enjoy cleaning the guts out -- so gross!" With little time to take a breath, I continued to ramble a mile a minute.

It was as if Dad was seeing me for the first time in years. He was listening and interested in what I was saying. In between the fun-loving banter about the camping expedition, Dad kept asking the same question to the point it was hard to ignore, "What have you been doing? How have I not noticed this? You look amazing, kiddo."

How could he not notice, when we, as a family, had been through some big changes over the last few months? Our meals alone were different. Our days of fast-food takeout were non-existent. At first, when Mom and I planned our summer adventure, it was our little secret (and Momo's too!), but now? Even Joey recognized the harsh reality that things would no longer be the same. Was Dad that wrapped up in his work that he hadn't noticed me at all?

Today's talk was one of the first and the longest that I'd had with Dad in a long time. I couldn't remember the last time I poured out my heart as I talked to him. Our talk gave him a chance to look and listen and notice how I had changed.

And if Dad could see a change, then others would too. What would I say when people asked? I didn't even know how to respond to Dad. I was certain no one would care about the details, the day-to-day progressive changes in my habits. Even as I went back and re-read my journal entries, even the worst of days didn't seem that bad.

I must have fallen a hundred times today while roller-skating . . . Messed up today when I ate too many of those keto peanut butter no-bake cookies . . . Can't believe how much energy I have; I can even keep up with Hudson! . . . I love my new swimsuit and walking on the sand at the beach . . . I'm missing Hannah and Chelsea. It stinks they spend their summers out of state . . . Wonder if anyone will notice or ask why I'm not shoveling a ton of junk food into my mouth.

My journal helped make me realize just how far I'd come. There were good days, filled with fun and wonder, but there were bad days too where I struggled. Especially in the beginning.

Dad was right; I changed. And, come fall, when school started again, it would no longer be a secret. Anyone who knew me from Haven Hills would see the new me.

The sound of excited yipping freed me from my thoughts. Mom and Joey had returned with Harmony and Hudson. They struggled to unclip their leashes as the dogs strained to reach me. As soon as they were released, the dogs jumped all over me, nearly knocking me to the couch and covering me with kisses.

BECOMING MISS IZZY

As I wrestled both dogs, I heard Dad asking Mom, "Can you believe how good Lizzy looks? She won't tell me her little secret," he added, winking in my direction.

"Let's save that for another time," Mom replied, wrapping her arms around me as soon as the dogs freed me.

"Right now, I want to hear all about your week of camping with the Collins!"

After tightening her hug, she met my eyes with pride, saying, "Your dad is right. You look amazing."

17. The Stumble

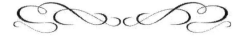

With only three weeks left of summer, I became more and more nervous about the adventure ending. *I'm anxious I won't be able to finish strong. I'm fearful I'll go back to the old bad habits. What if the new and improved me is just not good enough for everyone else?*

I tried reminding myself of the pros: *I lost twenty pounds. I have an abundance of energy. I'm trying new things and enjoying them. I sleep like a baby (no more tossing and turning like a fish out of water). I love the way I feel, and clothes look better on me now than before. So why would I want to sabotage myself since I'm so close to the finish line?*

When I voiced all my concerns to Mom, she assured me it was normal to feel this way. She had a way of encouraging me, redirecting my negative thoughts into positive ones; but despite her reassurance, I still felt I was on the verge of a major backslide of epic proportion. I had this little nagging voice inside my head.

It was more than willing to break all the rules. And, it found an opportunity the very next day.

Mom invited me to join her and Momo on a two-hour "road trip" to visit a friend who just settled into a nursing home. After she mentioned that Dad and Joey were going to a baseball game, I opted to stay home with the dogs, insisting they still needed their walk. I didn't want to raise suspicion.

With some reluctance, she agreed, making me promise to call her if I needed anything. She reminded me that Mrs. Collins was down the road should I need someone immediately.

As soon as everyone left the house, I made a beeline to the kitchen to see what I could find that would satisfy this craving. I was almost delirious. I wanted food -- lots and lots of food. I wasn't even sure why. I scurried around the kitchen in search of the perfect treat.

I found a bag of dark chocolate chips, so I made a batch of cookies. When they finished baking, I scarfed down the entire dozen, burning the roof of my mouth. Feeling just a tad bit guilty, I wrote in my journal as I lounged on the patio in Dad's hammock. Rather than run and chase Harmony and Hudson around the yard, I threw a ball from the confines of my comfy cocoon. I felt tired. The warm heat of the sun was making my eyes droop, and with the cool breezes lulling me deeper, I drifted asleep.

When I awoke, it was near lunchtime. Even though I wasn't too hungry, I was craving pizza. I had birthday money left over, so I called for delivery, telling the man on the phone not to skimp on the cheese. I found a coupon for fried cinnamon balls and added that to my order.

While waiting, I felt more guilt-ridden as I wrote in my journal. *Maybe I should have ordered a thin crust pizza with extra veggies. I wonder what Mom will say when she finds out about all of this.*

Harmony and Hudson signaled the pizza man's delivery before he got out of the car. Feeling grown and trying to absolve my anguish and guilt for what I was doing, I handed the driver twenty dollars and told him to keep the change. In no time, all that remained of the greased-stained boxes were a few ragged pieces of crust and a dusting of sugar. I devoured every one of the deep-fried sugar balls. Feeling like I had a bowling ball lodged in my gut, I waddled my way back to the hammock and fell into a fitful sugar-induced coma.

I didn't know what hurt more, my head or stomach. *Why did I do this to myself?* I couldn't remember the last time I'd felt this bad after eating something so good. My body wasn't used to this kind of food anymore. It couldn't handle it. Overcome with guilt and shame, I covered my face with my hands, hysterically sobbing into them.

18. Can I Love the New Me?

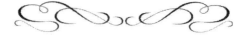

Mom was more disappointed than angry as she woke me from the hammock. I must have crashed and burned after filling myself with junk.

"Liz, get up. What happened to you?" she asked, her face warring between concern and disbelief. "Did you eat that whole pizza or did Harmony and Hudson help?" She picked up the empty box from the floor, the remaining pieces of crust gone. The dogs looked at us, little crumbs coating their muzzles.

I would have laughed at the scene had I not felt ashamed. "Mom, I am so sorry. I hate myself so much." the tears flowed, "Harmony and Hudson must have knocked the box over when I was sleeping to get at the remaining couple pieces of crust." I sank into the couch, my body wracked by sobs. "I don't know why I did this."

"It's just a pizza, Lizbeth. It's not the end of the world," she said, enveloping me in her arms and squeezing too tight for my flip-flopping stomach. "You put your body in shock, making it groggy. It's no big deal."

Even when I didn't think I had enough tears left in me, I pulled from the reserves; more began streaming down my face. I could barely talk, but between hiccups, I told Mom all about my binge-fest. "I feel so sick, too, which I deserve." I trailed off before adding, "I ruined everything! My entire summer adventures."

Although she kept calm and listened through my tears, I saw the resolve in her eyes before she stood, pulling me to my feet. She gripped the sides of my arms and gave me a little shake, drawing my gaze to meet hers. "The first thing you will do is stop your negative self-talk, Liz," she admonished. "You are not stupid. What you did does not make you a bad person. You're human. It is normal to feel upset. However, no one is perfect, and we all fall down. Everyone has setbacks. We all make mistakes or bad choices from time to time."

I was grateful that my mom understood and was patient and kind. And, her words packed enough of a punch I stopped wallowing in self-pity. Her encouraging nature always set me back on the right track, renewing my confidence.

As the end of our summer adventure was drawing near, I had that dreaded appointment with Dr. Adams. It worried me that my binge would set me back some, but I recovered well from my tailspin.

My transformation amazed Dr. Adams and his assistant. I had lost 25.5 pounds since my last visit. After some other tests, they gave me a remarkably clean bill of health.

All the changes from this summer made a big difference. I felt renewed, like a butterfly emerging from its cocoon. Like Mom, when she was my age, I was growing into myself. And I loved everything about it.

With middle school on the horizon, I felt more determined than ever to not only accept the new me but to love the new me, without condition.

19. From Hurt to Hope, to Happy

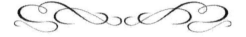

I t seemed like years had passed since the last time I'd locked myself in my room, devouring a whole pint of ice cream when feeling blue and down in the dumps. In reality, it was only several months ago before school let out for the summer, but during that time, I was heavy-hearted and even heavier in the waist. I worried about my weight on top of everything else life seemed to throw at me. Even the simplest things worried me and would reduce me to tears. And, because of the pain I felt, I never imagined I could one day be happy.

Not to sugar-coat life by saying everything was just "peachy-keen" now that my summer adventure was over . . . I still had my moments of despair. However, they were less frequent. And, I learned a few things about keeping hope and finding my happiness again.

It helped that Mom took her time introducing the health changes. She called them "mini-habits." She showed me a few books, but who wants to read self-help books? Maybe an adult, but not a kid! Mom deserved a lot of credit. She was sneaky because I didn't even realize I was adopting these new mini habits.

For example, one of the first mini habits she pushed at me was writing in my journal every day. Mom insisted that I write one sentence about how I felt at the start of the day. Then before going to bed, I had to write at least one thing I was grateful for. She said what I wrote was private, but I still had to flash my book at her to show I'd written at least one sentence.

Talk about a piece of cake. (Look at me, I still have that link to food in the back of my mind. LOL.) At first, I did the bare minimum. I covered one or two things I was feeling or thinking about. Soon it became helpful and freeing to write about everything I was feeling. On some days, I had pages of entries. After hearing the adults in my life go on and on about letting my emotions out, I never accomplished that until I started a journal. And, the part about writing what I was grateful for—it gave me the warm fuzzies and a better, hopeful outlook for the next day.

Mom also acquainted me with something she learned called "tapping." She showed me this after I had a meltdown one day. My brother was blaming me for the crappy snacks he had to eat, and Rachel bailed on me when we had plans to go to the pool that same afternoon.

This "tapping" Mom was doing looked ridiculous! And at first, I complained about it, but when I realized she meant business and would not take no for an answer, I took part. She instructed me to make a fist with one hand and tap the outside meaty part between my pinky and wrist with the fingers of my other hand. She called this the "karate chop" point. While tapping other various spots on my body, she told me to repeat after her, "Even though I am feeling rejected by everyone, I acknowledge my feelings and accept myself. Even though no one likes me and is blaming me for everything, that doesn't make me a bad person."

Huh? I felt stupid, but grateful that no one else was around to witness this strange event. We would have ended up in a padded cell. I was sure of that.

The funny thing, though, was that this "tapping" thing worked. I wasn't sure how or why, but after doing a couple of rounds, it felt like a weight lifted. It made me feel calmer and more assured of myself. I used this technique so much throughout my adventure that I would tap my collarbone without even thinking about it when I felt stressed. It didn't even matter if anyone was around who might have seen me doing it.

This summer, there were plenty of good things I accomplished. And, there were hard things to overcome. Even when I sometimes felt unprepared, I got comfortable with the mini habits. I used them often. And, you know the amazing thing about good habits? They allow you to find "your" happy.

PART III

ACCOMPLISHMENTS AND FUTURE COMMITMENTS

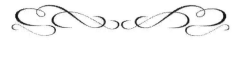

20. Yikes! Time to Start Middle School

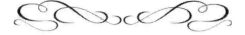

Although I was sad that Chelsea and Hannah weren't joining me at Ravenhurst Middle School, I was grateful I had Rachel. It would have been brutal starting the first day of school without at least one friend. I discovered Megan, and most of her mean squad would attend the same middle school. They cursed my luck!

Seeing how anxious I was the day before school started, Mom and Mrs. Collins planned a girl's day out for Rachel and me. We got mani-pedis and picked out the same vibrant tropical color to remind us of our adventurous summer. We rocked new hairstyles and tried on a million outfits, determined to win the school year. It was one of the best, carefree days we've had, the four of us laughing and bonding together.

The next morning, I stood before my mirror, modeling a new outfit. I couldn't believe my eyes! The image staring back at me was the girl I dreamed about several months earlier. I had transformed—like the ugly duckling that morphed into a beautiful swan. Seeing a healthy version of myself gave me confidence, providing me with a certain glowing radiance. I couldn't stop smiling.

When I joined Mom for breakfast, she gave me a pep talk on what to expect that day. She was the best person to talk to about this, considering she was a principal at a middle school in a neighboring district. If anyone knew what the first day of middle school was like for a kid, it was Mom.

She mentioned that today would be an orientation day. Since all sixth graders were new to the school, they would show us around. They would give us schedules, locker assignments, and the opportunity to meet our teachers and make new friends.

Just before I left home, Mom handed me a list and told me to read it on the ride to school. *First, be yourself. Just be you. You are good enough. Be confident, but don't be over the top. Have a positive attitude. Keep an open mind. Be curious and don't judge things too hastily. Plan to make mistakes and fail at some things. It's okay. Everyone will do it. It's your first attempt in learning. Don't over-think things and worry too much. Stay calm and adjust. Talk to at least three new kids. Find someone that looks like they could use a new friend and be kind to them. Take a risk and try something new. It's a little scary. However, who knows what it might lead? Remember your healthy min-habits from the summer. Balance your new routine with work and fun. Don't stress. Keep yourself bulletproof from stress.*

I found myself re-reading this list a couple of times during the day when I felt just the teeniest bit anxious. Last school year, I could blend in or hide behind my closest friends. Now? Standing out wasn't comfortable. I felt unprepared for all the attention. Treatment from the kids that knew me from Haven Hills was different. I was being complimented instead of ridiculed. It felt nice, but it was weird. I guess this was just something new that I would have to learn to get used to.

SUE ZOOK AND MARY LAZARSKI

Overall, it was a good first day of school, well, half-day technically. It was nice just having the sixth graders without the upper-grade kids there too. I only had about twenty other students in my homeroom I interacted with that first day. We had about two hundred and fifty in my grade alone. This would mean another possible five hundred kids between seventh and eighth grade.

Tomorrow should prove interesting when the hallways filled. I was also sure this would be the start of another adventure. *Get ready for some new trials and situations to learn from and enjoy the ride*, I said to myself.

21. When "Frenemies" Strike

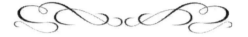

I accepted the fact that my two best friends were attending school at Maple Crest. What I couldn't take was that Megan was here, at Ravenhurst, torturing me with her evil presence.

I could breathe easier and even do a happy dance when I learned after yesterday's orientation that Megan and I had none of our classes together. And, with some miraculous luck, none of her friends did either. Unfortunately, Rachel had a different schedule from me too, but we committed to having each other's backs; or at least I thought at the time.

Mom told me that middle school was the perfect time to meet new people and make new friends. She mentioned that those I knew in elementary school might have changed, just like I did, and that it was okay to explore new interests and try new things.

She also warned me about something known as "frenemies." When I asked her what that meant, she explained, "You might find that someone who is a friend to your face and whom you consider a friend is, instead, a 'frenemy.' In fact, they are whispering behind your back or excluding you from activities."

It horrified me to think a friend would do something like that, but it seemed my grandma knew a thing or two about this "frenemy" topic.

After the first full day of school, Momo was practically bouncing in her seat with anticipation. Before we drove off, she grabbed my hands, begging me to tell her how my day was. "How was your first full day? Do you like your teachers? Did you make any new friends?" She threw question after question at me, without pause, causing me to laugh.

After answering each of her questions—*It was great! Yes, my teachers seem nice! I met a couple of new kids*—I noticed her smile wilted as her demeanor grew a bit more serious.

"What about Rachel? Did you see her today?" she asked, a frown etched on her face.

Surprised by this turn and a little curious at her concern, I answered, "Not since we went our separate ways at the door to our homerooms. We aren't in the same classes. I'll only get to see her at lunchtime, and on days we walk home together."

"Hmm," she huffed. "Well, I can't be too sure, but I saw Rachel hanging around Megan and her friends while I was waiting on you." She paused as if in thought. "It looked like they were making fun of a girl that looked an awful lot like Suzy if I recall. They were pointing and laughing at her."

Suzy? My mind was spinning. *Is she back?*

There was no way Rachel would hang out with someone as awful as Megan. I worried that she was being targeted. "Were they picking on Rachel as well?" I asked Momo, afraid of the answer.

"Didn't look like it. In fact, they all smiled and waved at each other as their rides picked them up. They seemed chummy enough," she replied.

Momo saw the stressed disbelief on my face and pulled over on the side of the road. She touched my cheek as a signal to turn my head. She looked me straight in the eyes. "I'm not telling you this to hurt you, honey. I want you to be aware and careful," she smiled, "Rachel may be trying out a new set of friends. It happens. Sometimes friends grow apart as they realize they want different things. I believe you'll know how to handle it if she is friends with Megan. Trust your instincts, Miss Izzy. You will know."

I wish I was more like Momo, although it was downright creepy the way she predicted things sometimes. That kind of intuition would be helpful in knowing how to handle difficult situations.

I sorted through my chaotic thoughts on the rest of the drive home. If Rachel turned into Megan, making fun of others all the time, I didn't think I could be friends with her. Maybe Rachel could see Megan for who she was and stand up to her? At least I hoped so.

And Suzy? Was that her that Momo saw? I wished it was her, and that she returned from out of town. Maybe this time around, I could be an influence and make a difference.

22. Forming a New Crew

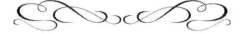

Mom and Momo were right about the whole "frenemy" thing. Deciding to give Rachel a chance, I called to see if she wanted to go to the park and exchange first-day-of-school gossip.

Unfortunately, when she answered, she said she couldn't talk long because she had plans to meet Megan at the mall. "I won't be walking to school with you," she said. "Maybe, I'll see you around."

The call ended abruptly. Her words were like a dagger to the heart. It seemed Rachel had chosen the dark side, the Darth Vader to my Luke Skywalker. Instead of wallowing in the hurt I was feeling, I would form my very own alliance. With much determination, I would make that happen.

The next day at school, I anticipated seeing Rachel and Megan together during lunch hour since all sixth graders ate at the same time. Without even glancing in their direction, I joined Jill and

Mia's table. I liked them the minute we met at orientation. We had an instant connection. They got along with everybody.

Unlike last year, we no longer had recess after lunch. We could choose where to sit, but we had to stick with that table for the duration of the hour. They did not permit table-hopping at this school. Although no one said this, I felt that the seats people chose that first week of school would become permanent seats for the rest of the year. As I scanned the room for familiar faces, I saw cliques of kids forming at tables, confirming my instinct. Megan and her regular squad were there, joined by their newest recruit, Rachel.

My eyes were drawn to a sparsely populated table. There were a couple of kids sitting there, off in their own worlds, none of them talking to each other. That's the table I spotted Suzy sitting. She looked a little different, taller, and perhaps somewhat slimmer, but there was no mistaking her. She came back!

When the lunch supervisor walked by my table, I waved, grabbing her attention. I pointed out Suzy's table, "I know a girl sitting there by herself. Would it be all right if I joined her?"

With a look of surprise, the supervisor smiled, "Sure, that's very nice of you."

A flashback of that horrible day last spring in the cafeteria at Haven Hills caused my knees to buckle as I meandered to the lonely table. However, no one seemed to notice me, including Suzy, as I slunk into the chair next to her.

"Hi, Suzy, it's me, Lizbeth Tanlin," I spoke, smiling. "It is so good to see you!"

Suzy's eyes widened in shocked recognition. "I thought I saw you walking to school alone this morning, but I wasn't sure," she paused, considering her words, "You look so different."

The last ten minutes of the lunch period flew by. As we talked, Suzy became more and more animated. She explained how things had not gone so well yesterday, being in the same homeroom as Megan. When she told her aunt and mom about that, they called the school. Because of the past problems Suzy had with Megan, the principal agreed that it was best they change her schedule. It would take a couple of days to get the new schedule in place, but as of Monday, Suzy would transfer to my homeroom. We were excited to exchange phone numbers so that we could talk over the weekend.

"Tomorrow let's sit together over there," I declared, pointing to the table of girls I sat with at the start of lunch. "I think you'll like Jill and Mia."

Suzy responded with a huge grin, saying, "Thank you, Liz, I'd love that!"

That lunch hour made my entire day. It was so heart-warming to see Suzy smile for once. And, I had a part in making that happen!

23. You Can Make a Difference

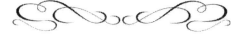

I t became easier and easier to be the new me. Although the changes I made in my healthy mini-habits changed how I looked on the outside, it seemed they had an even greater impact on how I felt on the inside. It's a little difficult to explain, but it felt like I was becoming more like Momo regarding *knowing* things. One thing I knew—I hated when I saw kids teasing other kids. And the hard-core bullies drove me crazy!

What was wrong with people? I experienced bullying as a bystander with Suzy. I witnessed it when mean kids picked on my brother. And, I was on the receiving end myself. I had to do something about it.

Suzy and I became instant friends after that first lunch period when I invited her to join the new friends I made and me. She confided in me, pouring out her heartache as she described her time at Haven Hills and life at home. Her parents divorced, and her mom suffered from nervous breakdowns. She wasn't able to take care of herself much less deal with what Suzy was going through at school. The incident in the cafeteria that spring was the last straw. Suzy couldn't take it anymore and begged her Aunt Judy to let her live with her although that came with its own hardships.

She was curious about how I had changed and wanted to learn about everything I knew. I felt guilty as I recounted my adventure. My hardest day was nothing compared to what she went through the past summer. However, it seemed she was eager to discover how she might start putting the healthier mini habits into action.

Suzy made light of the small transformation she made, but things were rough, and those changes didn't come by choice. Her parents' divorce had gotten ugly, and there was little money to accommodate the expenses. There wasn't much food in the house, so the weight she lost was because of that and performing various chores for her aunt.

Today we made a plan to work on a school assignment together, but then we took a break from it so that Suzy could let her emotions out. It thrilled me to know that she trusted me enough to unleash everything she was bottling up inside. I could relate to that since I used to do the same.

After her heart-wrenching tale, I wrapped my arms around her in a comforting hug. Through her tears, she smiled, and her spirit lifted.

"I was nervous about coming back and going to middle school," she whispered. "I hoped things would be different but knew in my heart they wouldn't be, but, then you showed up at my table." Suzy grabbed my pinky finger with hers, ready to seal a promise. "You changed my life, Lizbeth Tanlin. Let's promise to be friends forever. I want to be like you and help other kids too."

Amid our BFF hug-fest, an idea for the assigned community service project struck me like a lightning bolt. "We will help others!" I squealed with excitement. "I have an idea that will help a lot of kids, Suzy. With our service project, we will stop kids from getting bullied, just like we were. Together, we will change things and make a difference!"

24. When You Know You Matter Most

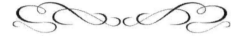

Over the next several weeks, Suzy and I worked tirelessly on our service project. We were developing a program to reduce bullying and make our school a safe and fun place for every kid.

Our school required every sixth-grade student to submit a service project idea. However, it was optional for students to enter their idea into the contest. For the contest, the staff chose one service project each year to put into action. I dreamed how amazing it would be if our project got picked.

At a school-wide assembly program, right before Thanksgiving break, they announced the winners of the best service project award. And, it was Suzy and I that won! It was our project that would be put into action!

Suzy and I were unable to contain our excitement as we walked through a sea of students, earning applause and high fives from our classmates. Teachers and our principal congratulated us too.

In the superintendent's speech, he mentioned how honored he was to fund such an amazing program. My face hurt as my smile grew bigger and bigger.

I could only imagine our program in action. We had steps in our plan to get students bullied away from the situation. We included a safe place for them to go where someone would listen to them tell their problem. Our program would have teachers, staff, and students be helpers or mentors. The helpers would provide support and make sure that kids picked on had a friend or two.

The program would provide fun lessons and training about how to prevent bullying. And, a support system would be available to every student throughout the school year. Our program would teach all students the skills to help them not be a bystander and know what to do, instead of to sit by and watch.

I was so caught up in the excitement that it took me a moment to realize I was in front of the entire school. I was astonished to see my peers smiling back at me. Well, at least most of them. Some didn't look too pleased, like Megan and her gaggle of wicked friends, but I took comfort in knowing that if they continued their mean ways, there would be a consequence to their actions.

After a final thunderous round of applause, Suzy and I made our way back to our seats in the bleachers. Out the corner of my eye, I saw frantic waving. When I turned towards the source, it surprised me to find Mom and Momo standing near the back wall. Mom blew kisses while Momo's hand shook her entire frame in a giant wave.

As soon as the assembly ended, I grabbed Suzy's hand and led her to the back to join my mom and grandma.

"I'm so happy to see you!" I gushed, throwing my arms around their waists. "I didn't know you were coming! How did you even know?"

Momo raised her brow intuitively. "Miss Izzy," she sassed, "You should know by now that I know *everything*."

I laughed. She sure did!

Mom held me at arm's length as to if to take in all of me. "I wouldn't have missed this for the world! I am so very proud of you." Her eyes glistened with tears. She glanced at Suzy, who stood behind me and smiled at her, saying, "So proud of both of you." She grabbed Suzy's hand and enveloped both of us in a hug.

Breaking free of the crushing embrace, I faced Momo whose smile could light the sky in the dead of night.

"You've come so far in the last six months, my special girl," she beamed. "It's remarkable how in tune you are to yourself. I admire everything you've done to help and inspire so many others."

As I reflected on her words of pride and encouragement, I felt amazing and was proud of myself. In just a few months of middle school, I had already proven that I mattered and was making a difference. Not just for myself, but for other people. Suzy and I were excited to get started and make our program come alive. We hoped all students would come to realize that the person who mattered most was the one that looked back at them in the mirror.

I found a poem that stuck with me. I wrote it down in my journal so I could remember to read it when I needed inspiration. The poem was originally called "The Man in the Glass" by Peter

Wimbrow, Sr. I changed a few words in it so that it would fit me better.

25. Changing from No to Now and Know

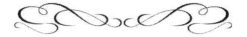

All things considered it's been an amazing adventure. It really seems like ages ago when I worried about every little thing and the word "No" filled so much of my daily life in the following ways.

No, you are not fat. You're my beautiful girl.

No, don't look so worried. You worry too much.

No, I'm not too full. Sure, I'll have seconds.

No, I can't handle the mean kids.

No, I'm not a good friend or sister when someone needs my help.

No, I'm not good enough.

Even as the school year ended, and the summer adventure began, I questioned myself and wondered whether I had it in me to make it through the journey. Looking back, that was a turning point. I had moved from focusing on "no" and looked at the "now" of a situation. With Mom's help, I could take those baby steps and be in the present and not worry about things too far ahead.

Focusing on what I could do right "now" got me through every situation; or at least most...

> I was in the *now* when I ate healthy meals each day.

> I stayed in the *now* by enjoying daily walks with Harmony and Hudson.

> I kept in the *now* by writing thoughts and feelings in my journal.

If I worried or schemed about something, I got myself in trouble. Like the time, I couldn't wait for Mom and Momo to go on their road trip so that I could binge on cookies, pizza, and deep-fried sugar-coated dough balls. I did not stay in the "now."

The funny thing about those types of situations -- I always learned something. I either gained more information that would help me in the future, or I learned a little more about myself. I was becoming more like Momo; I was starting to know things.

Momo calls it, "Listening to your intuition." I like to call it, "Being in the 'know.'"

Don't get me wrong. I didn't know everything and probably never would. However, I knew that if you paid more attention to what you did "know" and listened to it, life would get easier and easier to figure out. Make sense?

Compared to before, I was in the "know" about many things since my adventure.

I *know* myself better, and I *know* that I matter.

I *know* what foods give me energy and make me feel good and which ones don't.

I *know* about fitness, sleep, and other healthy habits.

I *know* family and other people who matter in my life.

I *know* stress and worry can make me sick.

I *know* about bullying, and other ways mean kids try to hurt you and what to do if it happens.

I *know* about gratitude and how it's important to find something you are grateful for every single day.

I *know* that life is an adventure we are all on, and experiencing it makes us who we are.

Like Mom, I finally grew into myself. And not just in the physical sense. I am confident. I am compassionate. I am a loyal friend and supporter. I became the person my grandma always called me, but I never truly understood it until now. I have become *Miss Izzy*.

Like Momo would say, "Do all you can, to be all you can be, and you will become the best possible you."

Sue's Acknowledgments

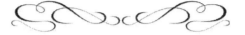

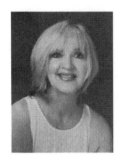

As long as I can remember, I had a nagging thought that someday, I would author a book. Then, at the sunset of my career after helping countless numbers of children and families on their adventure of life, I was faced with an even more nagging thought. *This can't be all there is. There are still so many people out there that I want to help. However, how will I make a difference as a retired educator?*

Several years into retirement, after dabbling in several programs to become a health and wellness entrepreneur, I surrendered to the idea of writing my first book. My hope and dream are that this book will not only entertain but inspire and help another countless number of children and families through the struggles and stresses encountered in the adventure of life.

There were a host of family members and friends, too numerous to name that encouraged me as I set out to begin writing. Dare I risk leaving someone off the list, let me say you know who you are. Thank you for the encouragement, inspiration, and support on my journey.

I do, however, want to mention several people who played a huge role in helping me make this book a reality.

First, I want to thank my daughter, Mary Lazarski. She truly gets me the most when it comes to understanding my passion for helping kids and families. She was a natural to call upon to collaborate on this effort. The "juice" you provided to the very first rough draft of the book brought life and freshness to Miss Izzy. I have thoroughly enjoyed working together on this project. In many respects, it felt like we were giving ourselves a "re-do" on our own life adventures. I hope this experience leads you to finish the first of many books inside you just waiting to be written. Don't wait as long as I did to make that happen! You owe it to so many to bless them with your gifts and talents.

Without the feedback I received on my first draft from my beta readers, I might not have had the courage or been inspired to take the next step. The 4 M's blew me away! With the attention to detail you provided in editing and the encouraging comments you made about how the book resonated with you and would be inspirational to young readers, you motivated me to keep going when I wanted to stop. Many thanks to all of you -- sister, Kelly Machak, Eillen Mauer, Cathy McDonald, and Alice Mical.

One of the hardest parts of the publishing process is turning it over to a professional editor or two. I searched for someone who would be tough on me. I wanted to learn as much as I could about making my writing better. I couldn't have asked for a better person than Nancy Pile from editor@zoowrite.com. I do not have the words left in me to express the debt of gratitude I have for everything she has taught me. I was shocked and amazed at the feedback she provided on my draft. It has been an honor and pleasure to work with her, and I look forward to continuing our partnership on future books in the Miss Izzy series. To my publishing editor and publisher, Dr. Melissa Caudle, from Absolute Author Publishing House, thank you for your words of wisdom and thank you for accepting my book into your publishing house making this book a reality.

105

Finally, although I said I didn't want to risk leaving anyone off the list who encouraged and supported me along the way, I would be remiss if I didn't mention by name two people who have been responsible for supporting me each week in my own health journey and post-retirement antics. Malina Chin, Vital Points Therapy, and Dr. Jeff Sima, Sima Chiropractic, thank you for helping me feel healthier and younger today than I did at the sunset of my career seven years ago. You're the best!

—

Mary's Acknowledgments

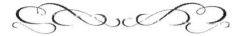

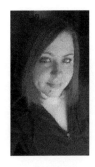I can't even describe the feeling you get when a book you've invested time, energy, heart, and soul into is finally published! There were so many that helped make this a reality, as my mother mentioned in her acknowledgments. However, my deepest gratitude goes to her. She's been my biggest cheerleader. I've always had a passion for writing. From writing my very first children's book about a lost sock while I was in high school, to writing the outline for my own YA dystopian fantasy novel just a couple of years ago, my mom was there, urging me to continue and expressing her enthusiasm to release my potential. I was thrilled when she asked me to collaborate on Miss Izzy's story, to develop the characters contained within and give them a voice and purpose. It awakened my desire to do more, and I think my mom knew that would happen all along. Thank you, Mom, for always being there, for always allowing me to express myself and for always encouraging me along the way.

I also wanted to thank my husband, Brian. After almost sixteen years together, he knows me more than I know myself. He knew how much I loved writing (and reading), so as a gift several years ago, he bought me my coveted laptop and Microsoft office so I could dive into writing my first book. Thank you, dear husband, for being my constant support, my confidant, my best friend, and the love of my life (even when I ignored you while my hands and mind were busy writing this book).

Lastly, I wanted to thank you, you, the wonderfully brilliant reader, that decided to pick up this book and give it a try. I hope you find this story valuable, relatable, and adventurous. After all, life is what you make it, and like Miss Izzy, make it great!

About the Authors

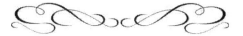

Sue Zook, Ed.D. served for over thirty-five years in public education as a teacher, mentor, building and district leader, and curriculum program developer. During that time, she helped thousands of children embrace a love for learning and a healthier lifestyle.

Since retiring as a district superintendent in 2012, Sue has continued to pursue her passion for helping young people. She is certified as a Health Coach and Wellness Educator by the Health Coach Institute and continues training and professional development for young people in the areas of health, wellness, and personal wellbeing.

Realizing that to help kids, Sue also has to help their parents. She has combined all her personal experience and professional expertise in a powerful solution to help children get rid of the struggles they are having with weight and other health, behavior and emotional problems that keep them from being their happiest and healthiest.

To learn more or schedule a complimentary health breakthrough session with Sue, visit her websites at:

nobesity4kids.com or healthcoachsue4u.com.

Email her at: info@healthcoachsue4u.com

BECOMING MISS IZZY

Mary Lazarski shares a passion for helping children deal with daily challenges and build self-esteem. Mary is an administrative assistant at a nonprofit drug and alcohol treatment center. She has over fifteen years of experience assisting both adult and teen clients. She lives with her devoted husband, Brian and their two cats, in Richmond, Illinois. In her spare time, she enjoys reading and writing fiction.

SUE ZOOK AND MARY LAZARSKI

BECOMING MISS IZZY

Made in the
USA
Columbia, SC